Cervical Spine Trauma

Cervical Spine Trauma

EVALUATION AND ACUTE MANAGEMENT

NORMAN E. McSWAIN, Jr., M.D.
Professor, Department of Surgery, Tulane University
School of Medicine, New Orleans, Louisiana

JORGE A. MARTINEZ, M.D.
Clinical Instructor, Tulane University
School of Medicine, New Orleans, Louisiana

GREGORY A. TIMBERLAKE, M.D.
CDR, MC, U.S. Navy, Department of Surgery,
U.S. Naval Hospital, San Diego, California

1989
THIEME MEDICAL PUBLISHERS, INC., New York
GEORG THIEME VERLAG, Stuttgart • New York

Thieme Medical Publishers, Inc.
381 Park Avenue South
New York, New York 10016

CERVICAL SPINE TRAUMA
Norman E. McSwain, Jr., Jorge E. Martinez, and Gregory A. Timberlake

Library of Congress Cataloging-in-Publication Data

McSwain, Norman E., 1937-
    Cervical spine trauma.

    1. Vertebrae, Cervical—Wounds and injuries.
2. Surgical emergencies. I. Martinez, Jorge A.
II. Timberlake, Gregory A. III. Title. [DNLM:
1. Cervical vertebrae—injuries. 2. Cervical Vertebrae—
radiography. WE 725 M478c]
RD531.M37 1988   617'.471   88-30079
ISBN 0-86577-299-1

Important note: Medicine is an ever-changing science. Research and clinical experience are continually broadening our knowledge, in particular our knowledge of proper treatment and drug therapy. Insofar as this book mentions any dosage or applications, readers may rest assured that the authors, editors, and publishers have made every effort to ensure that such references are strictly in accordance with the state of knowledge at the time of production of the book. Nevertheless, every user is requested to carefully examine the manufacturers' leaflets accompanying each drug to check on his own responsibility whether the dosage schedules recommended therein or the contraindications stated by the manufacturers differ from the statements made in the present book. Such examination is particularly important with drugs that are either rarely used or have been newly released on the market.

Some of the product names, patents, and registered designs referred to in this book are in fact registered trademarks or proprietary names even though specific reference to this fact is not always made in the text. Therefore, the appearance of a name without designation as proprietary is not to be construed as a representation by the publisher that it is in the public domain.

Printed in the United States of America.

5 4 3 2 1

TMP ISBN 0-86577-299-1
GTV ISBN 3-13-729101-7

To my daughter Merry McSwain, my mother
Mildred McSwain, and my sister May Ann "Bup"
Kightlinger. Thanks for your support, faith, and love.

Norman E. McSwain, Jr., M.D.

This book is dedicated to my parents, my brothers,
Gwendolyn, Krista, Nikolas, and Benjamin. Thanks
for your patience and faith in me.

Jorge A. Martinez, M.D.

Catherine Sue Timberlake, the love of my life,
without whose support I could not have come so far.

Gregory A. Timberlake, M.D.

Contents

Preface

One of the major challenges to the provider of initial care in the Emergency Department regarding the trauma patient is evaluation of the cervical spine. Immediate analysis of the cervical spine x-ray, determining need for immobilization of the cervical spine, or whether it is appropriate for orthopedic and neurosurgical consultation, and/or computed tomography scan or other specialized techniques is critical in the management of severely injured patients. It is important, therefore, for the physician working in the Emergency Department to be able to recognize problem films immediately. It is not necessarily important to establish a specific diagnosis. Approximately 15% of bony injuries to the cervical spine will not be detected on a cross-table lateral film; however, almost all unstable fractures will. For the physician caring for these patients, therefore, an understanding of three views is critical: cross-table lateral, anterior-posterior, and odontoid. It is to those films that this work is directed. This book is not intended to be a detailed analysis of the radiographic views of the cervical spine, nor is it aimed at the radiologist. Rather, it is addressed to the physician with day-to-day duties in the Emergency Department, including the emergency physician, surgeon, family practitioner, and the students of these disciplines—medical students, interns, and residents. This book also includes material on the acute management of such patients. As with the radiologic evaluations, this book does not provide in-depth management techniques, but addresses stabilization of the cervical spine injury until the appropriate specialist can arrive to provide definitive care. If such a specialist is not available, the packaging and stabilizing techniques can be used for transportation to the appropriate facility where such specialists are available.

The final chapter includes case studies so that after completion of the reading, the understanding of the techniques described can be applied. The case scenarios allow the readers to self-task and review the more subtle principles covered in the text.

Norman E. McSwain, Jr.
Jorge A. Martinez
Gregory A. Timberlake

ACKNOWLEDGMENTS

Without support staff no publication is possible: *Gae O. Decker-Garrad,* editing and criticism; *Winifred Hunter,* typing; *Vanessa Miller,* everything.

1

GREGORY A. TIMBERLAKE

Introduction

Recognition and management of cervical spine injuries in victims of trauma remain constant vital functions of the physician in the Emergency Department (ED). Many of these injuries may be subtle without associated spinal cord injury; in such cases the ED physician must make the diagnosis of a cervical spine injury in a timely fashion, without allowing any injury to the spinal cord to occur in the ED. If the patient already has a neurologic deficit, the ED physician does not necessarily need to make the diagnosis, but not allow any secondary insult to the patient that might worsen the deficit.

Adding to the stress of this responsibility is that the Emergency Medicine physician, or general surgeon, who first evaluates the trauma patient is often alone, without a radiologist, orthopedist, or neurosurgeon present to assist in initial evaluation of the roentgenograms. Every physician treating trauma patients in an ED must have a basic understanding of normal cervical spine anatomy, physiology, and radiology and, thus, be able to recognize symptoms, signs, or x-ray abnormalities indicative of a cervical spine injury. By having this knowledge, the physician treating the trauma patient initially will be able to prevent aggravation of existing injuries to the cervical spinal cord, as well as request appropriate specialty consultations to assist in further evaluation, diagnosis, and treatment of the cervical spine-injured patient.

Cervical spine injuries remain a major cause of morbidity and mortality in the United States. Between 8,000 and 12,000 surviving new spinal cord-injured patients are reported yearly, in addition to the already 200,000 quadriplegic or paraplegic patients alive in the United States today.[1,2] This translates to an incidence of 30 to 50 million per year.[3] The cost to society from these injuries is immense. It costs approximately $200,000 annually to rehabilitate a spinal cord-injured patient and $600,000 annually for the same nonrehabilitated patient to function in society as independently as possible. The overall cost to society to care for spinal cord-injured patients is $2 billion each year.[4,5] Unfortunately, only about 10% of spinal cord-injured patients are even admitted to rehabilitation facilities to retrain them in activities of daily living for a more productive and independent life.[6]

Cervical spine injury can result from both blunt and penetrating trauma (Table 1-1). Blunt trauma predominates and accounts for about 80% of injuries; motor vehicle accidents cause approximately 55% of all such injuries. In motor vehicle fatalities, there is a 21.1% incidence of cervical spine injury.[7] Penetrating trauma accounts for most of the remaining injuries, with gunshot wounds predominating. Iatrogenic injury, such as from chiropractic manipulation, is rare and accounts for less than 1% of cervical spine injuries. Unfortunately, not all cervical spine injuries are recognized initially in the ED and from 3.7% to 25% of patients with a cervical spine injury may incur paralysis or death by unwarranted manipulation of their head and neck in the ED.[4,8,9] Another reason early recognition of cervical spine injury is so important is because at least 5% of these patients will have injury in at least one other level.[10]

Rehabilitation services for the cervical spinal cord-injured patient are sadly lacking. Although the potential for rehabilitation is fairly good and rehabilitated patients cost society significantly less for their care, many

TABLE 1-1. **ETIOLOGY OF CERVICAL SPINE INJURY**

TYPE OF TRAUMA	%
Blunt	80
Motor vehicle accidents	45–55
Falls	10–20
Sports	5–10
Other	5
Penetrating	20
Gunshot wounds	5–10
Stab wounds	5
Impalement	1–2
Iatrogenic	<1

of these patients are discharged from the acute-care hospital without being rehabilitated. The prognosis and mortality of the cervical spinal cord-injured patient is also grim: for complete cervical spinal cord-injured patients, after one year the prognosis is 1% for total recovery, 7% for significant recovery, 59% with paralysis, and 34% die.[11] There is an important need for the physician managing the emergent trauma patient to understand the diagnosis and initial management of cervical spine injuries to prevent conversion from a neurologically intact patient to one who is quadriplegic or paraplegic.

REFERENCES

1. Bradford DS: Spinal instability: Orthopedic perspective and prevention. *Clin Neurosurg* 1980; 27:591–610.
2. Luce JM: Medical management of spinal cord injury. *Crit Care Med* 1985; 13:126–131.
3. Riggins RS, Kraus JF: The risk of neurologic damage with fractures of the vertebrae. *J Trauma* 1977; 17(2):126–133.
4. Young JS, Northrup NE: Statistical information pertaining to some of the most commonly asked questions about SCI. *Sci Dig* 1979; Spring: 111–127.
5. Hockberger RS, Doris PE: Spinal injury, in Rosen P (ed): *Emergency Medicine: Concepts and Clinical Practice.* St. Louis, CV Mosby Co, 1983, pp 289–330.
6. Committee on Trauma Research, National Research Council: Rehabilitation, in *Injury in America: A Continuing Public Health Problem.* Washington, DC, National Academy Press, 1985, pp 80–98.
7. Alker GJ Jr, Oh YS, Leslie EV, et al: Postmortem radiology of head and neck injuries in fatal traffic accidents. *Radiology* 1975; 114:611–617.
8. Bohlman HF: Acute fractures and dislocations of the cervical spine. *J Bone Joint Surg* 1979; 61-A:1119–1142.
9. Rogers WA: Fractures and dislocations of the cervical spine: An end result study. *J Bone Joint Surg* 1957; 39-A:341–376.
10. Calenott L, Chessare JW, Rogers LF, et al: Multiple level spinal injuries: Importance of early recognition. *Am J Roentgen* 1978; 130:665–669.
11. Foo D: Spinal cord injury and spinal shock. *Emerg Care Quart* 1985; 1:77–82.

GREGORY A. TIMBERLAKE

2

Anatomy and Physiology

A complete review of the complex anatomy and physiology of the cervical spine is beyond the scope of this book. A basic understanding of the normal anatomy and physiology, however, is critical so that the physician treating the trauma patient in the Emergency Department (ED) can recognize abnormal structure or function. This chapter will briefly review the normal anatomy and physiology of the cervical spine.

ANATOMY

Osteology

Man has seven cervical vertebrae. The first two are peculiar, the middle four typical, and the seventh is transitional. The cervical portion of the spine extends from the base of the skull to the thorax.

The typical cervical vertebrae (Fig. 2-1), as exemplified by the third, fourth, fifth, and sixth cervical vertebrae, is composed of an anterior body attached to a vertebral arch composed of two pedicles and two lamina. The body is equal in height anteriorly and posteriorly, but elongated from side-to-side, being about half as long transversely as sagittally. The vertebral body and vertebral arch surround the somewhat triangular-shaped vertebral foramen. The spinal cord lies within the vertebral canal formed by successive vertebral foramina.

The lamina are about the same height as the vertebral body, whereas

4

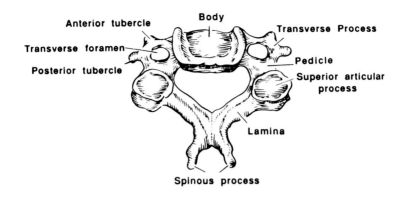

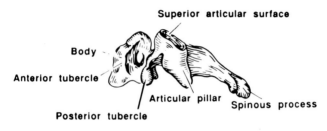

FIG. 2-1. A typical cervical vertebra and its parts seen from above (a) and the side (b).

the pedicles are shorter in height, giving rise to superior and inferior vertebral notches. With the adjacent vertebrae, these form the intervertebral foramen through which the spinal nerves exit the spinal canal.

Arising from the vertebral arch are several projections serving for articulation with other bones or for attachment of muscles. The transverse processes arise from the junction of the pedicles and laminae and contain the distinguishing feature of the cervical vertebrae, the foramen transversarium. It is through the foramen transversarium of the upper five or six cervical vertebrae that the vertebral arteries course. The transverse processes usually end in anterior and posterior tubercles; between these is a sulcus for the spinal nerve. The anterior tubercle of the sixth cervical vertebrae is prominent and is an important clinical landmark. Commonly called the "carotid tubercle," the common carotid artery lies in front of the tubercle and may be compressed against it to control hemorrhage distally.

Also arising from each pedicle-lamina junction are paired superior and inferior articular processes. These processes articulate with those of the vertebrae above and below to form the facet (apophyseal) joints. The facet joints are directed approximately 35° in an anterior direction with the inferior articular process of the vertebrae above laying superior and posterior to the superior articular process of the vertebrae below.

Finally, the spinous process projects posteriorly from the junction of the two lamina. The spinous process is typically short and angled inferiorly. The spinous process is frequently bifid as well.

The first cervical vertebrae (atlas) supports the skull and is atypical in that it does not have a body (Fig. 2-2). Instead, it is a ringlike structure composed of five equal areas. The anterior arch lies anterior to the odontoid process (dens) of C_2 and to the plane of the other cervical vertebral bodies. It has a prominent tubercle anteriorly for the attachment of muscles and posteriorly a facet for articulation with the dens. The paired lateral masses each have superior and inferior articular

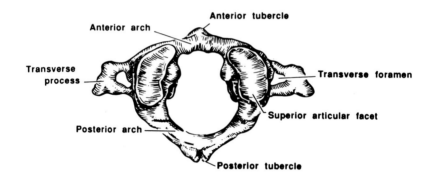

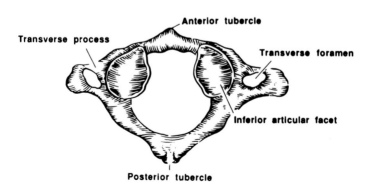

FIG. 2-2. The atlas (first cervical vertebra, C_1) seen from superior (a) and inferior (b) views.

facets. The upper facets articulate with the occipital condyles, whereas the inferior facets articulate with the superior articular facets of C_2. Also projecting from the lateral masses are the long and prominent transverse processes, which act as levers to help rotate the atlas (C_1). Finally, medially on each lateral mass a tubercle serves as a point of attachment of the transverse ligament of C_1. The right and left halves of the posterior arch are flattened from above downwards. Just posterior to the lateral masses, each half of the posterior arch has a groove over which the vertebral artery passes after it traverses the transverse foramen in the atlas. The atlas does not have a spinous process; instead, a posterior tubercle arises at the juncture of the right and left halves of the posterior arch.

The axis (C_2), the second cervical vertebrae, is another atypical cervical vertebrae. It is depicted graphically in Fig. 2-3. Projecting superiorly from the upper part of the body of C_2 is the dens or odontoid process. The dens articulates with the anterior arch of the atlas (C_1) above and is constricted at its base, where it is supported by the transverse ligament of the atlas. The paired superior articular facets are large, weight-bearing, and arise from the body and pedicles. As a result of this anterior placement of the superior articular facets, the second cervical nerve emerges posterior to this synovial joint (instead of anterior to it) and does not groove the transverse process that, thus, has only one tubercle. One further important anatomic feature of C_2 is that its vertebral foramen is smaller and rounder than that of C_1.

The seventh cervical vertebrae (C_7) is transitional between the typical cervical vertebrae and thoracic vertebrae. As such, its body is heavier and it has a long and unusual nonbifid spinous process. This prominent spinous process accounts for the vertebrae's alternate name, "vertebrae prominens." The transverse foramen are usually small and transmit only small veins. Occasionally, there is an additional rib(s) attaching to C_7, the so-called cervical ribs.

Although many anomalies of the cervical spine may occur, three are more common in the adult of which the ED physician must be aware. Occasionally, the occiput and atlas may be fused. Similarly, the axis and third cervical vertebrae (C_3) may also, and perhaps more commonly, be fused. Finally, as noted earlier, there may be cervical ribs associated with the seventh cervical vertebrae.

In children, knowledge of development of the vertebrae is important for the ED physician. Without an understanding of normal embryology and development, the physician caring for the injured child will be unable to discern normal developmental changes from fractures on roentgenograms.

The vertebral column develops around the notochord, the original

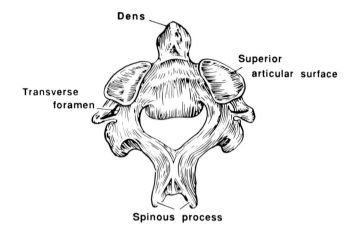

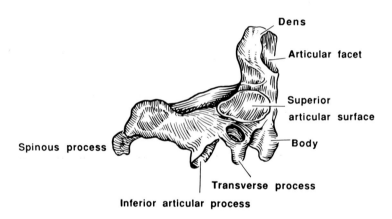

FIG. 2-3. The axis (second cervical vertebra, C_2) seen from superior (a) and lateral (b) views.

longitudinal skeleton of vertebrates. The notochord originates from mesoderm of the segmental mesodermal somites and is, itself, segmental. That portion of the notochord within the vertebral body disappears gradually, whereas the portion of the notochord between two vertebral bodies remains to form a portion of the intervertebral disc. After the vertebral body has formed, outgrowths extend posteriolaterally around the neural tube to form the neural arches. While this development is proceeding, chondrification centers develop in the body and spread so that by the third month of in utero development the entire vertebrae is cartilaginous. At about this time, three primary centers of ossification appear. One ossification center appears in the vertebral body, along with a center for each side of the arch. At birth, the typical cervical vertebrae consists of three pieces connected by cartilage. The neural arches normally fuse posteriorly by age one year, whereas the fusion of the two neural arches with the vertebral body usually occurs by the third year of life. Secondary ossification centers appear on the transverse processes, spinous process, and superior and inferior articular facets by puberty, along with ring epiphyses on the superior and inferior margins of the vertebral body. If the spinous process is bifid, a secondary ossification process develops on each tip. The secondary centers of ossification usually fuse by 25 years of age. It can be difficult to distinguish fractures from failure of fusion of ossification centers. If the ED physician is unsure whether a fracture or incomplete fusion is present, he should continue to protect the patient's spine until the radiographs of the cervical spine have been reviewed by someone with more experience and, if necessary, further x-ray studies have been obtained.

Ossification of the atypical cervical vertebrae, the atlas (C_1) and the axis (C_2), is also atypical. The atlas has one ossification center for each half of the posterior neural arch. These centers also give rise to the lateral parts with their articular surfaces. Ossification begins during intrauterine life, but the posterior arch does not fuse completely until about four years of age. A secondary ossification center for the posterior tubercle appears at about two years of age. Usually a single center for the anterior arch fuses with the centers for the posterior arch between the ages of seven and ten years. Occasionally, there may be two anterior centers of ossification, one on each side of the anterior tubercle, or the anterior arch may ossify by direct extension from the center on the posterior arch. Failure of any center to develop or of any two centers to fuse will result in a defect in the ring of C_1, which may be mistaken for a fracture.

The axis usually ossifies from five centers. These include paired centers for each half of the posterior neural arch, one for the lower body, and paired centers for the odontoid process (dens). The ossification centers for the dens are usually fused by the seventh month in utero so that at birth the axis appears to consist of four parts. The halves of the posterior arch fuse together with the lower body between ages three to six years. The dens begin to fuse with the lower body at about the same time, but complete ossification may not occur until 12 years of age. At times, incomplete fusion of the dens with the body may persist into adulthood. Where seen on roentgenograms, this appears as a thin, radiolucent, transverse stripe with sclerotic edges and may be mistaken for a fracture. Similarly, the secondary ossification center for the tip of the dens, resulting in the os terminale, which usually fuses with the rest of the dens by 12 years of age, may be visible radiographically and mistaken for a fracture as well. If this secondary ossification center fails to develop or unite with the body of the dens, a bulbous cleft dens may also occur (Fig. 2-4).

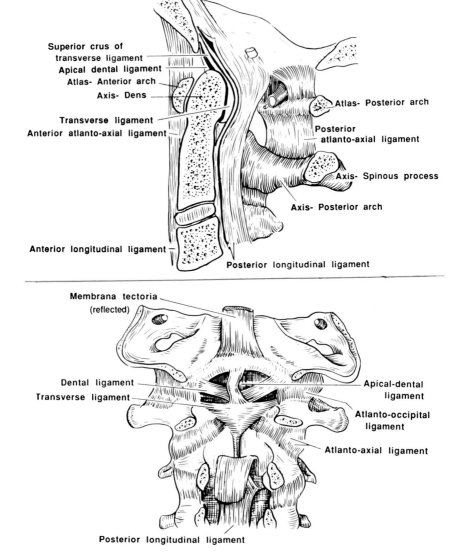

FIG. 2-4. The major ligaments of the cervicocranium seen schematically from the side in paramedian section (a), and from behind (b).

Intervertebral Discs

Between each pair of cervical vertebrae is an intervertebral disc, derived in part from the notochord, the primitive longitudinal skeleton of all vertebrates. In the cervical region, the discs are slightly greater in height anteriorly than posteriorly, which accounts for the normal curvature of the cervical spine. Each disc has two components, an outer "annulus fibrosis" and an inner "nucleus pulposus." The annulus is predominantly fibrocartilage and its fibers fan obliquely from one vertebral body to the next in concentric rings, thus giving elasticity to the annulus with compression and distraction forces. The nucleus pulposus is predominately mucoid with embedded reticular and collagen fibers. It has a high water content, which decreases when assuming the upright position and with advancing age. The nucleus is placed just slightly posterior to the center of the vertebral body and with both stress and age-related degeneration of the annulus, a portion of the nucleus pulposus may protrude posterolaterally through a defect in the annulus fibrosis.

Ligaments

Serving to join the vertebrae, provide stability, and allow limited movement, knowledge of the ligamentous anatomy is crucial to understanding the function of the cervical spine. Most complex is the region of the cervicocranium, that structural unit composed by the articulations of the skull to the atlas, and the atlas to the axis. Five synovial joints and four major ligaments are of importance in this region. The joints are the paired atlanto-occipital joints, paired atlantoaxial joints, and the joint between the dens and anterior arch of the atlas.

The most anterior major ligament is the anterior atlanto-occipital ligament extending from the superior surface of the anterior arch of the atlas to the anterior margin of the foramen magnum of the skull. The paired alar ligaments are the next most anterior major ligaments, running from each side of the apex of the dens superolaterally to the condyles of the occiput. These short, stout cords serve to hold the skull tightly to the axis and also check rotation of the cranium and atlas on the axis. The transverse ligament of the atlas is a strong, fibrous band extending between the medial tubercles of the lateral masses of the atlas. This ligament passes posterior to the dens and holds it against the anterior arch of the atlas, thus maintaining the normal relationship between these two bony structures. A synovial joint lies between the anterior aspect of the dens and arch of the atlas and between the posterior aspect of the dens and transverse atlantal ligaments. The most posterior major ligament is the tectorial membrane, a broad, strong, dense band that extends from the body of the axis to the inner surface of the occipital bone without attaching to the dens. These ligaments are illustrated in Fig. 2-5.

Several ligaments of lesser importance should also be noted in the cervicocranial region. The apical dental ligament runs from the tip of the dens to the anterior margin of the foramen magnum. The accessory atlantoaxial ligaments extend from the axis at the base of the dens, in the same direction as the alar ligaments, to each lateral mass of the atlas. Additionally, the anterior and posterior atlantoaxial ligaments and posterior atlanto-occipital ligaments warrant mention. Finally, it should be noted that weak superior and inferior bands run from the transverse atlantal ligament to the skull above and the body of the axis below, thus giving rise to the transverse atlantal ligament's alternate name, the cruciform ligament.

The ligaments for the remainder of the cervical spine may be thought of as in two groups: anterior and posterior (Fig. 2-6). The anterior ligaments attach to the bodies of the cervical vertebrae and serve to strengthen the fibrocartilaginous joint between two adjacent vertebrae. The anterior longitudinal ligament is a strong, wide band extending from the axis to the sacrum. Above the axis it becomes a thin cord, attaching to the occiput, and is, in part, continuous with the anterior altanto-occipital ligament. The anterior longitudinal ligament is attached closely to the annulus fibrosis of the intervertebral discs and end plates of the vertebral bodies, but less tightly to the concave vertebral bodies. This ligament is thickest and strongest anteriorly, less so anterolaterally, and serves to limit extension (dorsi-flexion) of the cervical spine.

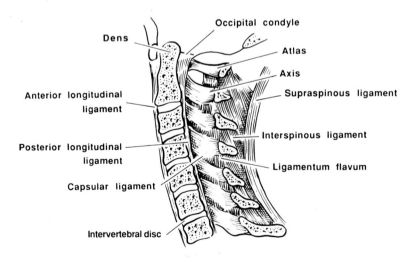

FIG. 2-5. Ligaments of the vertebral column.

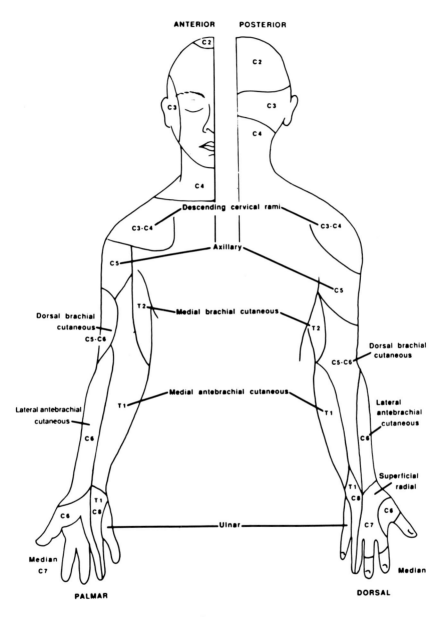

FIG. 2-6. Cervical nerve sensory dermatomes.

The posterior longitudinal ligament also courses from the axis to the sacrum, but along the posterior surface of the vertebral bodies. Its most superior extension is continuous with the tectorial membrane. Like the anterior longitudinal ligament, it is attached firmly to the ends of the vertebrae and intervertebral discs, but not to the center of the bodies. Flexion of the vertebral column is checked by this ligament.

The posterior group of ligaments attach to structures on the vertebral neural arches. The strongest and most important of the posterior group are the ligamentum flava, composed chiefly of elastic tissue. These thick, strong, paired ligaments arise from the anterior surface of the lamina of the superior vertebrae and course to the posterior superior edge of the lamina of the next inferior vertebrae. The ligamenta flava are separated in the midline (through which venous plexuses inside and outside the vertebral column communicate), and blend laterally into the capsular ligaments of the facet joints.

The facet joints have thin, loose capsules that connect to the articular surfaces of the adjacent vertebrae. These joint capsules are more lax in the cervical region than elsewhere in the spine to allow for the increased motion in this region.

Posterior to the ligamentum flavum in the cervical region is the ligamentum nuchae. This ligament extends from the external occipital protuberance to the spinous process of C_7, attaching to each spinous process, forming a septum between the posterior neck muscles. The two components to this ligament are: the interspinous ligament, a series of thin membranous structures passing from the base of one spinous process to the apex of the next; and the supraspinous ligament that joins the tips of the spinous processes. Although in many quadrapeds the ligamentum nuchae is a strong, thick elastic structure that aids the muscles in holding up their heavy head, in man these ligaments do not lend significant strength to the spinal column. These ligaments, particularly the interspinous ligament, are often sparse, or lacking, at one or more levels.

The intertransverse ligaments are located between the transverse processes of each cervical vertebrae. These ligaments add little to the strength of the vertebral column.

Spinal Cord

Within the vertebral canal formed by the successive vertebral foramen is the spinal cord with its meningeal coverings. This cylindrical structure, slightly flattened dorsoventrally, extends from the foramen magnum to about the level of the intervertebral disc between the first and second lumbar vertebrae in the adult. Corresponding to the greater nerve distribution to the limbs, the spinal cord is enlarged in the cervical and lumbar regions. The spinal cord occupies about 50% of the cervical vertebral foramen, the remainder being occupied by an epidural venous plexus, with associated fat and connective tissue, and the meninges of the spinal cord.

Three meninges cover the spinal cord. The outermost is the dura mater, a tough, thick, fibrous tube contiguous with the cranial dura mater at the foramen magnum and extending distally to the level of the third sacral vertebrae, and fixed caudally by the filum terminale to the coccyx. Lying closely applied to the spinal cord is the pia mater. The arachnoid mater, which is flimsy and attached to the pia by threads, is located in between. The space between the arachnoid and pia, filled with cerebrospinal fluid, is known as the subarachnoid space. The spinal cord is held in place by a series of dentate ligaments arising from the pia and attaching to the dura.

Arising from each segment of the spinal cord are the 31 pairs of spinal nerves, which are named segmentally: eight cervical, 12 thoracic, five lumbar, five sacral, and one coccygeal. Each peripheral nerve is formed from a dorsal (sensory) root and ventral (motor) root. The efferent ventral roots emerge from the apices of the anterior horns of gray matter, while the afferent dorsal roots converge on the apices of the posterior horns of gray matter. Running laterally from the spinal cord, the nerve roots are covered with pia mater as they cross the subarachnoid space and then successively are covered with arachnoid and dura mater. At the level of the intervertebral foramen, the dorsal root is swollen by the presence of a spinal ganglion. Just distal to this, the two nerve roots unite and mingle to emerge from the intervertebral foramen as a nerve trunk. The cervical nerves exit above the level of the adjacent vertebral body, except for C_8, which exits between the seventh cervical vertebrae and first thoracic vertebrae. Below this level, the nerves exit through the intervertebral foramen below the vertebral body.

VASCULATURE

Each vertebrae is supplied by paired segmental arteries. In the cervical region, these are derived from the vertebral arteries. Each artery gives off multiple branches that eventually supply the vertebral body and arch, anastomose with the vessels above and below, supply the tissue of the epidural space and meninges, and variably provide a portion of the arterial supply to the spinal cord.

The major route of arterial supply to the spinal cord, however, is through the paired posterior spinal arteries and single anterior spinal artery. The anterior spinal artery is formed from a root arising from each vertebral artery, which branches just before the junction of the vertebral arteries to form the basilar artery. The paired posterior spinal arteries arise as branches of the vertebral arteries or posterior inferior cerebellar arteries. The amount of blood flow supplied to these arteries from the vertebral arteries is sufficient only to supply the upper cervical spinal cord segments, so that these arteries are variably reinforced by branches of the segmental arteries to the vertebral bodies.

The venous drainage of the vertebral bodies and spinal cord parallels the arterial supply. In addition, both an internal and external vertebral plexus of valveless veins communicate through channels in the intervertebral foramina. In the cervical region, blood from the external vertebral venous plexus empties into the vertebral veins.

Soft Tissue Spaces

Lying just above the anterior longitudinal ligament in the neck is a soft tissue space known as the prevertebral space. It has two components, a retropharyngeal space and, below this, a retrotracheal space. These spaces are defined anteriorly by an air-tissue interface, which on roentgenography is ordinarily a sharp, distinct line. Note that the esophagus, which lies posterior to the trachea, is normally collapsed, and thus not ordinarily visible on cervical spine x-rays. Embedded in these tissues is a prevertebral fat pad that lies just above the anterior longitudinal ligament, which may be seen as a "fat stripe" on a lateral cervical roentgenogram in adults. Displacement of this line anteriorly may be the only indication of injury in some patients. Although commonly visualized in adults, the prevertebral fat stripe is seen less frequently in children.

Physiology

The normal function of the cervical spine and spinal cord is complex and only an outline of this function can be given here.

The vertebral column in the early embryo is "C"-shaped. By birth, the original anterior concavity of the cervical spine has become abolished. As the infant learns to hold its head up and sit up, the normal secondary posterior concave curve is established. This change is a compensation to the upright posture in man.

In general, mobility of the vertebral column is a result of the elasticity and compressibility of the intervertebral discs that allow limited motion of the vertebral bodies upon one another in any direction. The stability of the vertebral column results from the presence of the normal curves and ligaments that bind the vertebrae together. The type of motion allowed between any two vertebrae is related primarily to the position of the synovial joints between them.

In the cervical region, the atlanto-occipital joint primarily permits flexion and extension and allows limited lateral bending. Primarily, the atlantoaxial joints allow rotation. The normal atlanto-odontoid relationship is maintained in neutral position, flexion, and extension by the transverse atlantal ligament. This interval in the adult normally does not exceed 3 mm on a lateral radiograph.[1] At the remainder of the cervical intervertebral joints, flexion, extension, lateral bending, and some rotation are allowed by the structure of the joints and ligaments. Fielding[2] has studied, cineradiographically, the motion of the cervical vertebrae and the reader is referred to his work for further details.

In infants and children, the same basic movements of the cervical vertebral joints are present. At the atlantoaxial joint, however, a greater degree of motion in flexion and extension is allowed by the infant's and child's normal physiologic ligamentous laxity. For example, the interval between the anterior arch of the atlas and odontoid process, normally not exceeding 3 mm as in the adult, may vary from 2 to 5 mm, with the maximal separation occurring with flexion.[1]

Similarly, physiologic anterior displacement of the axis on C_3 or C_3 on C_4 may occur in up to one quarter of children to age eight years.[3] In a child who has sustained trauma that might have affected the neck, the finding that one vertebra has an anterior position compared to its subadjacent one may give rise to concern that a fracture, dislocation, or both are present. If no other stigmata of injury are present, this concern should be alleviated by demonstration of a normal relationship of the posterior laminar lines of C_1 through C_3.[4,5]

In the ED, demonstration of normal function of the spinal cord traversing the cervical region is implied by demonstration of normal sensory, motor, and reflex functions of the body parts. In the midcervical region of the spinal cord, the spino-thalamic tract, which conveys fibers for pain and temperature sense, is the anterior white matter. The posterior columns conveying touch, position, and vibration sensation are distributed through the anterior, lateral, and posterior white matter. The main descending fibers for motor function are in the lateral corticospinal tract located in the lateral white matter.

As noted earlier, the segmental spinal nerves arising from the spinal cord are mixed motor and sensory nerves formed by the junction of the afferent dorsal and efferent ventral nerve roots. As a result, sensation over the body has a segmental distribution, described as dermatomes (see Fig. 4-1). Similarly, the segmental innervation of the body's voluntary

TABLE 2-1. **SPINAL CORD MYOTOMAL INNERVATION**

LEVEL OF LESION	MUSCLER INNERVATED BY NERVE ROOT ABOVE	RESULTING LOSS OF FUNCTION
C_4	Diaphragm	Spontaneous breathing
C_5	Trapezius	Shrugging of shoulders
C_6	Biceps, brachioradialis	Flexion at elbow
C_7	Triceps	Extension at elbow
C_8 to T_1	Flexor digitorum profundus and superficialis	Flexion of fingers
T_1 to T_{12}	Intercostals; abdominals	Accessory respiration; tighten abdominal wall

Cervical nerve root supply for major muscle groups and resulting loss of function in case of injury. Only the major spinal roots are listed; a specific muscle is frequently supplied by multiple spinal roots. Variation is not uncommon.

TABLE 2-2. **CERVICAL NERVE ROOT LEVELS FOR TENDON REFLEX EXAMINATION**

LEVELS OF LESION (AT OR ABOVE)	RESULTING LOSS OF REFLEX
C_6	Biceps
C_7	Triceps
L_4	Patellar
S_1	Achilles

musculature and normal deep tendon reflexes are shown in Tables 2-1 and 2-2.

The reader is advised to consult standard anatomic and physiologic texts for further details of the anatomy and physiology of this most important area.

REFERENCES

1. Locke GR, Gardner JI, Van Epps EF: Atlas-dens interval (ADI) in children. *Am J Roentgen* 1966; 97(1):135–140.
2. Fielding JW: Cineroentgenography of the normal cervical spine. *J Bone Joint Surg* 1957; 39-A(6):1280–1288.

3. Cattell HS, Filtzer DL: Pseudosubluxation and other normal variations of the cervical spine in children. *J Bone Joint Surg* 1965; 47-A(7):1295–1309.

4. Swischuk LE: Anterior displacement of C_2 in children: Physiologic or pathologic? *Radiology* 1977; 122:759–763.

5. Harris JH Jr, Edeiken-Monroe B: The normal cervical spine, in *The Radiology of Acute Cervical Spine Trauma*, 2e. Baltimore, Williams and Wilkins, 1987:pp 1–44.

3

NORMAN E. McSWAIN, JR.

Kinematics of Trauma

INTRODUCTION

For many years, the Halstedian philosophy that history is 90% of the diagnosis of any condition has been a part of the general assessment of the patient. Only recently has the idea been applied by practitioners of emergency medicine to blunt trauma patients. It is particularly applicable with injuries to the cervical spine from deceleration or compression trauma because these patients can be apparently without injury, but the potential for paraplegia or quadriplegia lurks with only a slight twist of the head or hyperflexion of the cervical spine. It is extremely critical for the practitioner of the post-crash phase of vehicular trauma to be knowledgeable of the crash phase, so that potential injuries can be managed without increasing the injury to the patient.

The three phases of any crash or deceleration injury are the pre-crash, crash, and post-crash components. The pre-crash phase of cervical spine injuries can be influenced by the practitioner who encourages such safety precautions as mandatory seatbelt use by every occupant in any vehicle. The post-crash phase (in which practitioners spend most of their time) is that of patient care. One has little influence over the crash phase, except prevention; however, without understanding the dynamics, many injuries will be missed for prolonged lengths of time. The longer such injuries remain undetected, the greater the possibility of associated complications. Resuscitation frequently requires that possible injuries be anticipated and protected while more critical components are being addressed. As has been emphasized continually by the American College of Surgeons, Committee on Trauma, Advanced Trauma Life Support Course, airway management is done with protection of the cervical spine. When should the cervical spine be protected? It is in understanding the kinematics of trauma that such a question can be answered appropriately.

To understand the mechanisms of injury, certain physical laws must be reviewed and their applications taken into account as the practitioner mentally reconstructs the accident to define what parts of the body were bent or twisted to produce possible or probable injury patterns of the patient.

PHYSICAL LAWS

Conservation of Energy

Newton's Second Law of Motion states that energy can be neither created nor destroyed, but can be changed in form. When energy (motion) has been imparted to a body, it begins to move through time and space. For the body to stop moving, the energy it contains in its momentum must be absorbed. When the front part of an automobile comes to a sudden halt as it impacts an immovable object, the rear of the automobile continues to have energy and forward motion. For that motion to be absorbed, the car bends along its frame (Fig. 3-1). If the front of the car has stopped by sudden impact with an immovable object, the torso continues forward. The head impacts the dash or windshield. The frame of the patient bends just as the frame of the automobile does. The "frame" of the patient is the spine, most likely the cervical spine. This can produce a fracture or it can produce extension/flexion/rotation injuries without fracture, but with muscle ligament or tendon rupture.

Momentum

Newton's First Law of Motion states that the body in motion or body at rest will remain in that state until acted upon by some outside force. When an automobile, motorcycle, bicycle, or person falling from a height has been set into motion, it continues in that fashion until some force changes its direction or absorbs its energy. A biker over a motorcross jump does not stop its forward motion simply because the bike has left contact with the ground (Fig. 3-2). The bike continues to move through time and space until something stops the forward

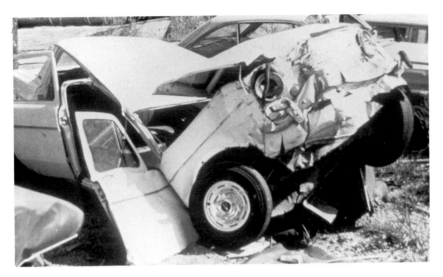

FIG. 3-1. Energy must be absorbed before motion ceases. The front of the pictured automobile stopped against a dirt embankment; the rear did not stop until its energy was absorbed by bending of the frame.

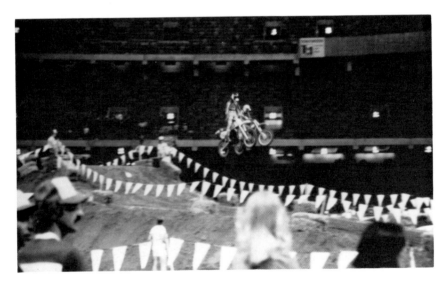

FIG. 3-2. Loss of driving force does not produce cessation of motion. When energy is established, it continues until absorbed. The bike and its rider do not stop because contact with the ground has been lost. The unrestrained occupant of an automobile does not stop its motion simply because the automobile hits an immovable object and stops. The occupant has the same forward motion of the biker and does not stop until the dash, windshield, or steering column/wheel are contacted.

motion. So it is with the occupant of an automobile or the rider on a bicycle or motorcycle. When the vehicle has imparted speed and energy to the occupant, that speed and energy remain. Should the car, motorcycle, or bicycle come to a sudden halt, the unrestrained occupant continues to move forward at the same rate of speed until something slows the motion (e.g., the windshield, in the case of a car; a tree, the struck automobile, or the asphalt, in the case of a motorcyclist or bicyclist).

The spinal column is similar to a stack of 24 building blocks placed one on top of the other with an 8-pound bowling ball on top. The stack has been further compromised by the curves developed in the alignment of the spine when homo sapiens evolved from four-legged posture to an upright carriage (Fig. 3-3). The pelvic tilt, the fatty protuberance on the anterior wall, and muscular laxity tend to further exaggerate these curves. In the cervical spine, the extra weight of the head and eccentric position of the center of gravity with regard to the

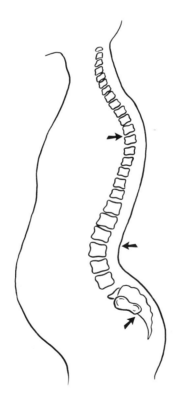

FIG. 3-3   Extra fat and poor posture exaggerate the "S"-shaped curves of the spine.

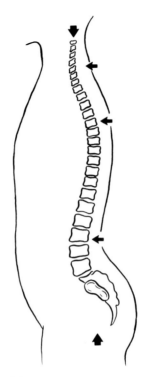

FIG. 3-4. Compression of the spine in the cephalad/caudad direction bends the spine wherever curves are already present. The tendency is to break one's "S."

head produce a force that distracts, compresses, or rotates this pile of blocks much more so than if they were alone.

A person falling from a height has the same kind of momentum. When the ground is struck by the feet, the torso and head continue to move until the energy is absorbed. The spine bends most at the greatest angle of its "S," breaking the S. Landing feet first, the lumbar and thoracic vertebrae at T_{12}, L_1, and L_2 are extremely vulnerable (Fig. 3-4). When landing head first, the cervical spine at either C_1, C_2, C_5, or C_6 is at greatest risk. When a person falls from a height and lands on his feet, the head does not stop its momentum and can continue either in a hyperflexion or hyperextension mode tearing tendons and ligaments, resulting in either a dislocation or partial dislocation of facet. It can come down and impact with the chest. A female may bear the "lipstick sign" on the breast as an important diagnostic finding (Fig. 3-5).

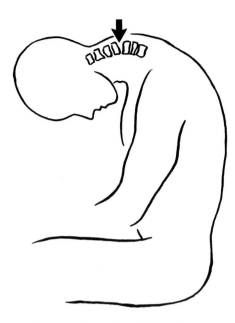

FIG. 3-5. When the downward motion of the torso stops upon impact with the ground after a fall, the momentum of the head hyperflexes or hyperextends the cervical spine. Lipstick marks on the breast or chest indicate such a motion has occurred.

Kinetic Energy

Kinetic energy is equal to one-half mass times velocity squared, $KE = M/2 \times V^2$, where: M = mass and V = velocity. As can be seen by this formula, the amount of potential energy in a moving object is more dependent upon its velocity than its mass. Doubling the speed of an automobile or motorcycle does not simply double the potential energy of the occupant, but squares it. A car impacting an immovable object at 40 mph, therefore, has much more energy contained in the impact than if the impact were half as great at 20 mph. More energy must be absorbed, therefore, more damage occurs to the occupant than in a slower speed impact.

Force

Force is equal to mass times acceleration (deceleration). Force is the amount of energy the moving object has to be absorbed on impact. Because acceleration and deceleration are measured in "G" forces, a moderately low-rate-of-speed collision of only 30 G of deceleration with a 150-pound occupant would produce 4500 pounds of force. This energy must be absorbed before the body will stop. The deceleration forces on frontal impact to the body, or the acceleration forces on lateral- or rear-impact collisions, must be considered as the practitioner evaluates the patient to try to determine the type and severity of the injuries involved.

COLLISIONS

There are five types of collisions, as well as composite crashes, automobiles can undergo and two types of motorcycle or bicycle collisions. Each of these different types of collisions produces a predictable impact pattern that the practitioner can use in determining possible injuries.

The three components to each collision are: the vehicular collision, the occupant collision, and the organ collision.

Frontal-Impact Collision

When a car and occupant traveling in a forward direction through time and space suddenly impact an immovable object, the car stops but the unrestrained occupant does not. The occupant continues forward until the body is brought to rest by impacting some part of the inside of the car, or by being ejected from the car and impacting some object surrounding the car or bike. If the head is the lead point of the human missile, it may impact the windshield, a pillar, roof, or dash of the car. The momentum of the thorax continues and its energy must be absorbed either by impacting something on its own or by absorption—bending or crushing the cervical spine.

Depending on the point of impact of the skull on the external object and relationship of the impact point to the cervical spine, the neck may be hyperextended, hyperflexed, or compressed (Fig. 3-6). This introduces the second factor that gives the practitioner a clue to the extent and type of injury to the patient. The first is the type of collision and its speed; the second is damage to the occupant. Injury to the occupant's head or face (any injury above the clavicle) indicates the impact point was in such a position that the momentum of the torso could well have been absorbed on the cervical spine. These patients should have the spine immobilized until x-ray evidence indicates no fracture exists. The same holds true with a helmeted victim. The helmet, if crushed, scratched, or otherwise damaged following a collision, is the indicator of significant energy absorption by the cervical spine (Fig. 3-7).

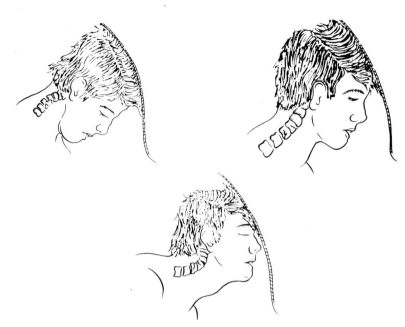

FIG. 3-6. During impact with the windshield, dash, or steering column, the neck must absorb much of the energy of the impact. Depending on the position of the torso, head, and impacted object, the head will be hyperextended, hyperflexed, or compressed.

Lateral-Impact Collision

In a lateral-impact collision, a car crossing an intersection is hit in the side by another vehicle. Additional energy and a new direction of motion are suddenly imparted to both the car and occupant. As in any crash, the components of the body that are in direct contact with the car rapidly gain this new motion and energy. Parts of the body not in contact with the car do not gain the new energy and direction until such forces are transmitted to them by their attachments to the body parts or body components connected to the car.

In a lateral crash, the door usually impacts the lateral side of the torso, whereas the head is not impacted. The torso begins its new lateral motion and the head continues to move forward. The next structure to move laterally is the neck; the head is last to begin its lateral motion. The eccentrically placed center of gravity of the head produces not only lateral bending toward the side of the impact, but rotation of the face toward that side as well (Figs. 3-8 and 3-9). It is this double motion that inflicts damage to the cervical spine with a greater frequency than seen

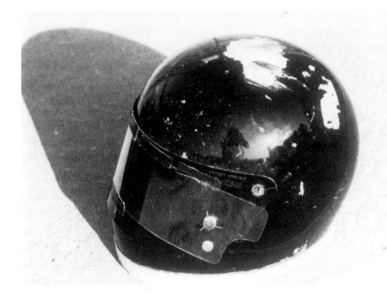

FIG. 3-7. Facial, scalp, or head injury alerts the examiner to the possibility of energy exchange involving the neck. Because the structures are protected by a good helmet, appreciation of the amount of energy exchange must come from an evaluation or (at minimum) a description of the helmet.

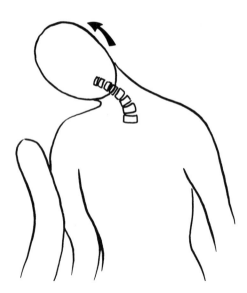

FIG. 3-8. During lateral impact the torso is accelerated out from under the head. Only the ligaments and muscular attachments prevent total spinal separation. Severe angulation of the spine, however, results along with distraction, especially on the side opposite the impact. Bony injuries are more common during lateral than rear collisions.

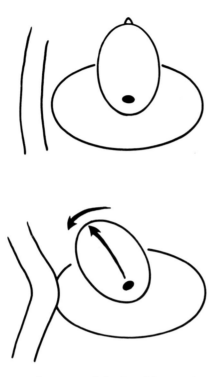

FIG. 3-9. The center of gravity of the head is anterior to the pivot point of the skull and neck. This tends to rotate the face forward to the impact point while pushing the neck away from it. The resultant forces to the vertebrae are a combination of rotation and angulation.

in rear-impact collisions. This can result in either lateral compression fractures or rotational injuries with torn ligaments, unilateral jumped facets, and/or dislocation.

Rear-Impact Collision

A rear-impact collision will accelerate all parts of the body equally if the occupant has maintained the headrest in the upright position, minimizing the possibility of cervical spine hyperextension. If the head rest is pushed down so that the spine hyperextends across it, however, sharp angulation of the spine occurs across the top of the headrest (Fig. 3-10). Significant ligamentous and tendon injury will result as well as compression of the posterior elements. Because no rotation is involved in this type of head motion, fractures and dislocations are seen less frequently than in lateral impacts.

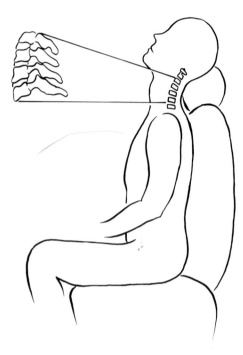

FIG. 3-10.   A rear-impact collision pushes forward all components of the body that are in contact with the car. If the head restraint is not high enough to contact the posterior skull, severe angulation of the neck occurs.

Rotational-Impact Collision

Front-quarter panel impacts cause rotational impacts; front-quarter or rear-quarter panel impacts produce rotation around the object. This produces a combination of both head-on and lateral-impact injuries (or rear- and lateral-impact injuries) (Fig. 3-11).

Rollover Collision

Rollovers produce a multitude of injuries as the unrestrained occupant careens from one surface of the inside of the passenger compartment to another. At each impact, energy exchange and absorption are transmitted to the tissues with subsequent damage.

Restraints

If the vehicular occupants slow at the same rate as the vehicle and are prevented from impacting the dash or the steering column in a frontal or combined frontal-rear impact, the automobile itself will absorb the

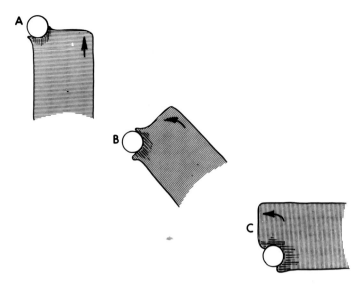

FIG. 3-11. Many accidents occur with the point of impact not directly in front of the center of gravity of the automobile. The center of gravity tends to push in the direction of motion. The result is rotation of the vehicle around the impact point, which produces a combination of motions to the occupant. The injury patterns produced are both frontal and lateral.

energy with minimal transmission to the occupant. In a lateral impact, if the occupant is propelled to the side at the same time as the car, the only damage to the occupant will be by compartment intrusion. The unrestrained occupant receives both intrusion and movement impact.

Restraining systems such as automobile safety belts do exactly this. By watching NASCAR, SCCA, and CART races, one can appreciate that violent energy exchanges can be almost completely absorbed by the vehicle with very little being transferred to the occupant. The three-point system available in the modern automobile is almost as effective as the five- or six-point restraining systems in the race car. The comfort factors of inertia reels, seats moved close to the dash or steering wheel, and the lack of passenger compartment integrity (built into the racing vehicle) can be supplemented by the addition of air bags. Air bags are no replacement for safety belts, but are additional safety factors.

COMPOSITE CRASHES

Additional information the examiner must acquire is where and in which car the injured occupant was sitting. Most two-car collisions in-

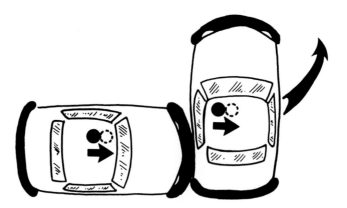

FIG. 3-12. Almost every collision between two vehicles produces different motions in each car. To determine what types of force (and, therefore, what type of injury patterns) are produced, the EMT (or patient) must be questioned to determine the impact point of the vehicle.

volve different points of impact on each car (Fig. 3-12). The examiner must know exactly where the patient was sitting upon impact, as well as what part of the patient's car was impacted (and its speed), to estimate the pattern and severity of injuries that would be expected. The probable speed (or energy absorption) can be judged by the amount of damage to the automobile.

MOTORCYCLE/BICYCLE CRASHES

On a bicycle or motorcycle, the occupant can impact his own vehicle, but more likely will be ejected and impact either the object his vehicle hit, a stationary object on the side of the road such as a parked car or tree, or the asphalt itself. If the examiner has enough information to reconstruct the flight of the patient and his point of impact with the ground or other object, a much better prediction can be made as to the severity and type of injury to be expected. Without this information, however, the examiner must assume the presence of spinal fracture until a Roentgenograph can prove otherwise.

BIOMECHANICS

As the head stops its forward motion in a collision and the torso continues its forward motion, the changing relationships of each individual vertebra to its adjacent vertebra must be considered.

Daffner et al.[1] have recently demonstrated that in frontal collisions with impact speeds greater than 35 mph, there is a 10% incidence of cervical-spine fractures, 3% thoracic, and 4% lumbar. Two thirds of the cervical fractures were hyperflexion on the driver's side, and one third was hyperextension. On the passenger side there were 6% cervical, 1% lumbar, and no thoracic fractures.

Hyperflexion Injury

Direct compressive force into the bodies of the cervical vertebra crushes the body and fractures the cortex. Because the posterior spinal elements provide additional support, if the head is flexed at the time of impact or the impact point is located in such a position as to produce hyperflexion, more compression will be on the anterior aspect of the vertebra producing a wedge-type fracture.

Hyperflexion itself tends to direct the compressive forces into the vertebral body (particularly the anterior part of the vertebral body), whereas the posterior components, both of the ring and spinal processes, tend to separate. Disruption of the intraspinous ligament, or one of the ligaments supporting the lamina or arch, tends to make the cephalad-caudad positioning of the cervical vertebra unstable resulting in dislocation (Fig. 3-13).

Dislocation compromises the canal lumen and, as such, impinges

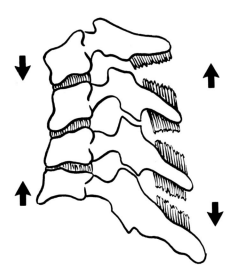

FIG. 3-13. Hyperflexion injuries compress the anterior column and separate the posterior column. This tends to compress the anterior part of the vertebral body and separate the spinous processes.

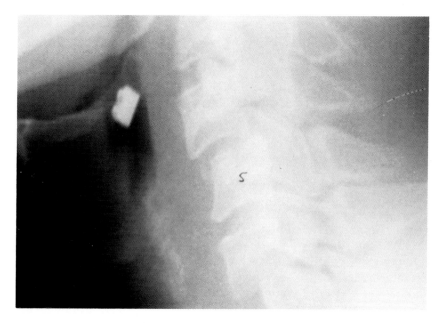

FIG. 3-14. Dislocation of one vertebra on another reduces the size of the spinal canal. In the cervical region this space is only slightly larger than the cord itself. Any compromise will compress the cord and produce edema, both of which lead to anoxia of the nerve fibers.

upon the spinal cord (Fig. 3-14). Such pressure may be only minimal and produce bruising or it can be more severe and produce extensive hemorrhage, ischemia, or both.

Hyperflexion is associated with opening of the facets and, in some cases, movement of the vertebral body forward. These joints tend to close, locking rather than returning to their original position (Fig. 3-15).

Hyperextension Injury

Depending upon the pivot point of hyperextension injury, either the anterior spinous ligament ruptures or posterior elements are compressed. This condition may produce more pain but less likelihood of an unstable situation than the hyperflexion injury.

The comparative strength of the posterior versus that of the anterior ligaments will determine which component (or both) will release. The vector forces compress the posterior elements, which act as a fulcum. The anterior longitudinal ligament stretches to retain the position of the

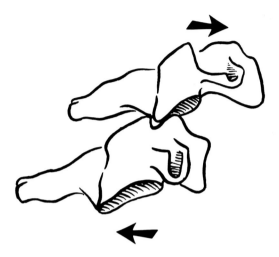

FIG. 3-15. Facets that override those just below will be trapped "over the lip" and cannot return to their original position.

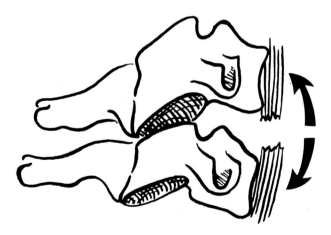

FIG. 3-16. Hyperextension of the vertebra compresses the posterior column and separates the anterior one. The compression can produce fractures of the posterior elements. The anterior column is separated. If the separation is severe enough, the ligamentum flavum will be stretched or torn.

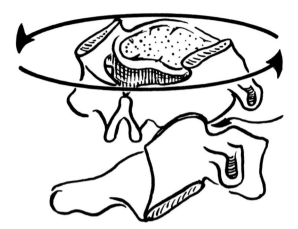

FIG. 3-17. When rotation is combined with lateral flexion, the facet on only one side can separate and overlap producing a unilateral locked facet.

vertebral body (Fig. 3-16). An avulsion fracture of the anterior body may be the key to the diagnosis of such a fracture.

Rotation

If disruption of the ligaments is associated with rotary movement of one vertebral body on another, unilateral locked facet or compromise of the cervical canal can result (Fig. 3-17).

Rotation of the upper vertebra on the one just beneath it compresses one pair of facets tightly together while separating the other two. In its pure form, the position is likely to be maintained, but when combined with lateral flexion or with hyperextension or hyperflexion dislocation, overriding and, therefore, locked facets become a real possibility.

REFERENCE

1. Daffner RH, Deeb ZI, Lupetin AR, et al: Patterns of high speed impact injuries in motor vehicle occupants. *J Trauma* 1988; 28(4):498–501.

4

GREGORY A. TIMBERLAKE

Assessment of Patients with Cervical Spine Injuries

The multiply traumatized patient brought to the Emergency Department (ED) presents a diagnostic and therapeutic challenge to the attending physician. All significant injuries, many of which are occult, must be identified and treated expeditiously. At the same time, no further harm must be incurred to the patient, either because of ill-advised diagnostic or therapeutic maneuvers or because of lack of awareness of injuries. As the injuries are identified, they must be addressed in order of severity following the guidelines of first salvaging life, then limb, and only then cosmesis.

To achieve the highest possible rate of salvage, the physician in the ED must have a plan of action. We recommend the physician adhere to the precept(s) of the Advanced Trauma Life Support (ATLS) course of the American College of Surgeons (ACS).[1] In this model, the initial evaluation and treatment of the trauma victim is divided into five stages (Table 4-1).

The first stage is a primary survey for life-threatening injuries following the "A-B-C-D-E" mnemonic shown in Table 4-2. Patency of the patient's airway is ensured while maintaining cervical spine control to prevent secondary injury. Often, merely opening the airway using the jaw-thrust or chin-lift technique may be sufficient, but oropharyngeal, nasopharyngeal, or endotracheal intubation should be performed if needed. If the patient with a potential cervical spine injury is not breathing and emergency airway access is required, cricothyroidotomy

TABLE 4–1. **FIVE STAGES OF INITIAL EVALUATION AND TREATMENT OF THE TRAUMA VICTIM**

Primary survey for life-threatening injuries
Resuscitation of vital functions
Secondary survey for injuries
Definitive care
Stabilization and transportation

must be considered. When the airway is assured, attention is directed to "B" for breathing. The physician must make sure there is no impediment to the exchange of oxygen and carbon dioxide through the lungs. Specifically, the physician must quickly evaluate the patient for the presence of tension pneumothorax, open pneumothorax, or other mechanical barriers to effective pulmonary gas exchange and ameliorate any that may be found.

Subsequent to this, the patient's circulatory status is assessed. This assessment is undertaken from two points of view. First, is the cardiac pump action sufficient? Second, is there exsanguinating external hemorrhage present? Signs of adequate cardiac pump function can be assessed with a few simple maneuvers including feeling the pulse, assessing the capillary refill time, and evaluating signs of end-organ perfusion. The pulse is assessed for rate, regularity, and fullness. As a general rule, if only the carotid artery pulse can be felt, the patient's systolic blood pressure is 60 torr; if the femoral artery pulse is palpable, the systolic blood pressure is about 70 torr; if the radial artery pulse is palpable, the patient's systolic blood pressure is at least 80 torr. The capillary refill test is performed by compressing the nailbed of one of the patient's fingers with the examiner's thumb and determining the length of time for the normal pink color to return to the nailbed after release of pressure. Usually, the time interval is no more than two seconds. A prolonged capillary refill time implies diminished perfusion

TABLE 4–2. **FIVE PHASES OF THE PRIMARY SURVEY**

A – Airway management, with cervical spine control
B – Breathing
C – Circulation, with hemorrhage control
D – Disability, from neurologic injury
E – Exposure

of the vascular bed. This test may also be performed on the thenar or hypothenar eminence, over a toe nailbed, or on the patient's earlobe. Signs of inadequate end-organ perfusion, which may be seen during the primary surgery, include anxiety, cool, clammy skin, complaints of thirst, and restlessness.

"D" in this mnemonic stands for disability and is used to remind the examining physician that central nervous system injury, when unrecognized and thus delayed or untreated, is a common form of long-term disability in the multiply injured patient. It also serves as another cross-check for adequate cerebral oxygenation. To evaluate for these injuries during the primary survey, the physician must assess the patient's level of consciousness (using some type of rapid, simple scale such as the "AVPU" method [Table 4-3]) and the size and reactivity of the patient's pupils.

Finally, "E" stands for exposure of the patient—all of the patient's clothing must be removed. Because this must be done without causing further injury, in the multiple-trauma patient the patient's clothes are usually cut off.

The second stage of the initial assessment is resuscitation of the patient's vital functions. Reliable venous access with large bore cannulas must be obtained in at least two locations and infusions of appropriate fluids and blood should be initiated. Supplemental oxygen is added, if not already begun, to keep the patient's PaO_2 at approximately 100 torr. An electrocardiogram monitor should be attached to the patient. A nasogastric tube and Foley urinary bladder catheter should also be placed at this time, unless contraindicated by the patient's injuries. Placement of a nasogastric tube initially is contraindicated if a cribiform plate fracture is suspected. Signs of this injury include midface fractures and cerebrospinal fluid rhinorrhea (a bloody discharge from the nares with a positive "halo test" when a drop is applied to a piece of filter paper). If a cribiform plate fracture is suspected, an orogastric tube should be placed instead. Placement of a Foley catheter is contraindicated if the patient is found to have blood at the urethral

---

TABLE 4-3. **THE AVPU METHOD FOR EVALUATING LEVEL OF CONSCIOUSNESS**

A – Awake and alert
V – Responds to verbal stimuli
P – Responds to painful stimuli only
U – Unresponsive to external stimuli

meatus, a scrotal hematoma, a high-riding prostate on rectal examination, or complaints of inability to urinate. Further urologic evaluation is required before a Foley catheter can be inserted.

When immediately life-threatening injuries have been found (if present) and treated, and resuscitation has begun, the third phase of the initial evaluation, the secondary survey, is begun. This phase involves a complete, head-to-toe physical examination of the patient. At this point, a more thorough evaluation of the patient's neurologic status should be made. This should include use of a reliable, objective scale for assessing the patient such as the Glasgow Coma Scale (Table 4-4). The goal of this phase is not only to find all injuries present, but to ensure that no new life-threatening injuries have appeared or recurred despite therapy. In concert with this, a patient history should be obtained. Although this should be as complete as possible, the minimal amount of information necessary to care for the patient is contained in an "AMPLE" medical history, as shown in Table 4-5. The patient's tetanus immunization status should also be ascertained.

The fourth phase of the initial assessment follows and is termed "definitive care." Here the appropriate specialists and therapies for the

TABLE 4–4. **GLASGOW COMA SCALE**

FUNCTION	POINTS
Eyes open	
Not at all	1
To pain	2
To verbal stimulation	3
Spontaneously	4
Best verbal response	
None	1
Incomprehensible sounds	2
Inappropriate	3
Disoriented and converses	4
Oriented and converses	5
Best motor response	
None	1
Extensor posture (decerebrate)	2
Flexor posture (decorticate)	3
Complex flexion	4
Localizes pain	5
Obeys	6

Individual scores are given for each function. The total score is the sum of the three functions and may range from 3 to 15.

TABLE 4-5. **"AMPLE" MEDICAL HISTORY**

A – Allergies
M– Medications currently being taken by the patient
P – Past illnesses
L – Last meal
E – Events preceding the injury

patient's injuries are marshalled and treatment is begun. This phase is followed by the fifth and final stage, stabilization and transportation, as the patient is readied for transfer from the ED to the next level of care. This may involve an intrahospital transfer to the operating room, intensive care unit, or ward, or an interhospital transfer to a regional trauma center.

Although the risk of a cervical spine injury being present is acknowledged in the primary survey with the admonition that the airway must be made patent while control of the spine is maintained, the actual evaluation for cervical spine injury belongs in the secondary survey. During the secondary survey, as the neck is examined and a neurologic examination is performed, important historic details should be obtained from the patient, paramedical personnel, police, or witnesses to the accident. The mechanism of injury must be elicited in detail. For example, for the victim of a motor vehicle accident, the ED physician should ascertain whether or not the accident was multivehicular, and if so, the angle(s) of incidence, speed of the vehicle(s), deformities of the car, steering wheel, windshield, or dashboard; whether the patient was the driver or a passenger; where the patient was seated in the car; whether seatbelts were worn; whether the patient was ejected from the car; etc. A history of neck or neurologic injury should also be obtained. Symptoms of cervical spine injury, as shown in Table 4-6, include a history of loss of consciousness, neck pain or stiffness, weakness, or parasthesia. Signs pointing to a cervical spine injury include unconsciousness, head or maxillofacial injuries, paralysis or paresis, parasthesia, hematoma, crepitance, or abnormal bony contour, and wounds to the neck with penetrating trauma. A trauma patient who is unconscious or has an altered mental status, even if caused by alcohol or drugs, should be presumed to have a cervical spine injury and have the cervical spine protected until the physical and radiologic evaluation ensure injury is not present. The ED physician should, likewise, be suspicious that a patient with injuries from the level of the clavicles cranially may have a cervical spine injury as well. Finally, the physician must be aware that

TABLE 4–6. **SYMPTOMS AND SIGNS SUGGESTIVE OF CERVICAL SPINE INJURY**

SYMPTOMS

History of unconsciousness
History of fall of more than three times patient's height
History of high-speed motor vehicle accident
Neck pain or stiffness
Weakness
Parasthesia

SIGNS

Unconsciousness
Head injury
Maxillofacial injury
Paralysis or paresis
Parasthesia
Cervical hematoma or ecchymosis
Cervical crepitance or abnormal bony contour
Cervical tenderness
Penetrating cervical trauma
Altered mental status caused by drugs or alcohol

in some multiple-trauma patients, the pain from other injuries such as a femur fracture or clouding of the sensorium by alcohol or other drugs, may obscure the symptoms of a cervical spine injury without neurologic deficit. If the unwary physician does not question the patient carefully about neck complaints, no matter how slight, and protect the spine until certain that an injury is not present, a cervical spine injury may be missed with potentially disastrous results for the patient. Most of the reports of painless cervical spine fractures in the literature[2-4] may, perhaps, be explained by this mechanism.

Part of the evaluation of all multiple-trauma victims is a complete neurologic examination. In the primary survey, as mentioned earlier, this examination is limited to assessment of the papillary responses and the level of consciousness or coma. During the secondary survey, a more complete and detailed neurologic examination must be performed and documented. Again, the patient's level of consciousness must be determined and changes noted. All 12 cranial nerves must be tested, not only those determining the pupillary responses (CN II, III, IV, VI). Testing of the olfactory nerve (CN I) is often neglected; however, it should be checked because anosmia may be a significant disability

to the patient and may even be a hazard to the patient in certain oc-
cupations.

Cerebellar function is difficult to test formally early in patient management, but any nystagmus, abnormal motion of the extremities, or
difficulty with finger-to-nose testing (if possible to perform) should be
noted.

A sensory examination is performed, with care being taken to evaluate at least the sensations of light touch, pain, and either vibration
or proprioception. If necessary to map out subtle changes, temperature sense can also be tested. Light touch sensation should be tested
using a camel's hair brush or a few wipes of cotton from the end of
a cotton-tipped applicator. Pain sensation is usually evaluated by pin-
prick. The practice of using a straight pin, pin-wheel, or safety pin kept
pinned to the physician's coat is mentioned only to be condemned. In
today's society, with fear of AIDS and hepatitis, a new, sterile, hypo-
dermic needle should be used for each patient.

It is important that a full sensory examination be carried out, particularly if a deficit is found. This is particularly crucial if the deficit is
in the lower cervical to upper thoracic region. The reason for this can
be seen by referring to the dermatome chart in Fig. 4-1. If care is not
taken, an examiner who notes a loss of sensation below the level of the
patient's clavicles may incorrectly ascribe this to an injury at the thoracic level of the spinal cord, when further, more detailed examination
may instead indicate the level of the lesion to be cervical.

Testing of motor function should be the next step in evaluation. The
major muscle groups (as defined in Table 4-7) are evaluated for tone
and strength. Any flaccidity or abnormal rigidity should be noted. The
strength of voluntary muscular activity in these groups should be noted
on a scale of 0 to 5, with 0 representing complete lack of strength and
5 normal strength, as shown in Table 4-8.[5]

Deep tendon reflexes (DTRs) may also be evaluated at this time
(Table 4-9). The DTRs most commonly checked include the triceps,
biceps, brachioradialias, quadriceps ("knee-jerk") and gastrocnemius-
soleus ("ankle jerk"). Normal brisk DTR responses indicate the reflex
arc through the spinal cord is intact and functioning. Absent tendon
reflexes imply that the reflex arc has been interrupted. Unusually brisk
or sustained tendon reflexes are seen with damage of descending
fascilatory tracts in the spinal cord.

One of the most important distinctions the initial examiner can
make, at least for patient prognosis, is whether the spinal cord lesion is
complete or incomplete. This classification determines whether there
is total loss of sensory, motor, reflex, and sympathetic activity below
the presumed level of injury, or if a portion of any of these functions

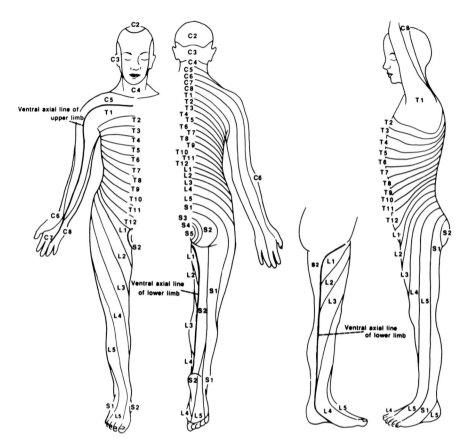

FIG. 4-1.   Sensory dermatome chart.

persist. Depending on the pattern of lost and retained activity, several spinal cord syndromes can be described. Prognostically, findings indicating an incomplete spinal lesion are important because the chance of useful functional recovery is more likely in such cases. To diagnose an incomplete lesion, the attending physician must give special attention to the genital reflexes and the phenomenon of sacral sparing. The genital reflexes include the anal wink, bulbucavernous reflex, and penile erection (priaprism). The anal wink is elicited when gentle stroking of the skin in the perianal region produces contraction of the anus. Loss of this reflex and loss of voluntary contraction of the anal sphincter during rectal examination, coupled with the absence of motor control below the upper extremities, indicate complete motor paralysis is present. The bulbocavernosis reflex is stimulated by either a pull on the

TABLE 4–7. **MYODERMAL INNERVATION OF THE MAJOR MUSCLE GROUPS**

MUSCLE GROUP	SPINAL ROOT	MAIN ACTION
Trapezius	C_3, C_3	Shoulder elevation
Diaphragm	C_4	Respiration
Deltoid	C_5	Arm abduction
Biceps, brachioradialis	C_5, C_5	Forearm flexion
Extensor carpi radialis	C_6	Wrist extension
Flexor carpi radialis	C_6, C_7	Wrist flexion
Triceps	C_7	Forearm extension
Flexor digitorum profundis and superficialis	C_8	Finger flexors
Interossei	T_1	Finger abduction and adduction
Intercostals	T_4	Muscles of accessory respiration
Abdominals	T_{10}	Tighten abdominal wall
Iliopsoas	L_1, L_2	Thigh flexion
Quadriceps	L_3, L_4	Leg extension
Tibialis anterior	L_4	Foot dorsiflexion
Extensor hallucis longus	L_5	Great toe dorsiflexion
Gluteus maximus	L_5, S_1	Thigh extension
Semitendinosus, semimembranosus, biceps femoris (hamstrings)	S_1	Leg flexion
Soleus, gastrocnemius, flexor digitorum longus, flexor hallucis longus	S_1, S_2	Foot and toe plantar flexion
Anal sphincter, bladder	S_2, S_3, S_4	Anal sphincter tone, urinary retention

TABLE 4–8. **GRADING OF VOLUNTARY MUSCULAR ACTIVITY**

POINT	FUNCTION
0	No movement
1	Visible muscle contraction
2	Movement of the joint with gravity eliminated
3	Antigravity power
4	Slight weakness
5	Normal power

Adapted from: Medical Research Council: *Aids to the Examination of the Peripheral Nervous System. Memorandum No. 45.* London: Her Majesty's Stationery Office, 1976.

TABLE 4–9. **NERVE ROOT SUPPLY FOR DEEP TENDON REFLEX INNERVATION**

SPINAL ROOT	PERIPHERAL NERVE INNERVATION	REFLEX
C_5–C_6	Musculocutaneous nerve	Biceps jerk
C_7–C_8	Radial nerve	Triceps jerk
C_5–C_6	Musculocutaneous nerve	Radial jerk
L_2–L_4	Femoral nerve	Knee jerk
S_1	Sciatic and tibial nerves	Ankle jerk

urethral catheter, which stimulates the trigone of the bladder, or by a gentle pinch of the glans penis, resulting in a reflex contraction of the anal sphincter around the examiner's finger. This reflex is important because if the patient is not in "spinal shock" (discussed below) and there is no sensory or motor sparing, but this reflex is present, then a complete spinal cord lesion is present. Sacral sparing is defined as the presence of normal perianal sensation. Again, finding sacral sparing or that the patient retains any ability to discriminate between a sharp and dull stimulus, indicates an incomplete spinal cord lesion. With either of these findings, the prognosis for eventual recovery is improved.

Although it is covered in greater detail in Chapter 6, a guide to the neurologic examination of the cervical spine-injured patient would be incomplete without a brief discussion of "spinal shock." This syndrome is seen with a complete loss of all distal DTRs and cutaneous reflexes after a complete spinal cord injury. All voluntary muscles are paralyzed and all sensation is lost. Also, all autonomic activity is lost below the level of injury. Piloerection and sweating are thus absent and bowel, bladder, and sexual functioning are disturbed. The genital reflexes, described earlier, are abolished as well. As a consequence of loss of sympathetic tone below the level of injury, the blood pressure may drop, although usually not below 90 torr systolic. A hallmark of "spinal shock" that helps differentiate it from hemorrhagic, cardiogenic, septic, or anaphylactic shock is that in association with the diminished blood pressure, there is a reflex bradycardia, not a compensating tachycardia, and a warm and pink skin. Because "spinal shock" is only seen in patients with complete (or dense, but incomplete) spinal cord lesions, its duration may have prognostic significance.

Having decided, based upon the history and physical examination, that a cervical spine injury may be present, the examining physician must obtain the appropriate radiologic studies. Much controversy exists over how many and what roentgenograms should be obtained. Currently, the debate centers on how extensive the basic cervical spine x-ray series should be. On one hand, a technically adequate cross-table lateral cervical spine roentgenogram should allow a diagnosis or suspicion of significant injury in up to 90% of patients.[6,7] On the other hand, some have advocated routine use of computed tomography (CT) scan for all suspected spine injuries.[8] No one test, or even series of tests, is likely to achieve 100% specificity and sensitivity in this area. Also, management of other life-threatening injuries may necessitate a less than "full" cervical spine series. For example, the patient who is hemodynamically unstable and requires expeditious transfer to the operating room cannot be delayed in the Radiology Suite while multiple views of the cervical spine are obtained. In such a case it may be sufficient to obtain a technically adequate, portable, cross-table lateral cervical spine roentgenogram and then proceed to surgery with the patient's cervical spine still protected. If this view is completely normal, the anesthesiologist, for example, may be able to intubate the patient's airway with less trepitation. If any abnormalities are seen in the film, the anesthesiologist may need to modify the techniques and control the airway with nasotracheal intubation, or have a cricothyroidotomy or tracheostomy performed by the surgeon.

Assuming the patient is clinically stable, however, the debate over the basic series involves only whether three or five views of the cervical spine, if normal, are sufficient to "clear" the cervical spine of injury. The most important view is the cross-table lateral roentgenogram of the neck, which should demonstrate most, but not all, unstable cervical spine injuries. An example of a cross-table lateral x-ray cleared by the radiologist, but later found to have a significant dislocation, is seen in Fig. 4-2. The open-mouth odontoid view is necessary to provide further details on the cervicocranium, whereas the anterior-posterior view provides added details on the lower cervical vertebrae. Although all agree these three views are mandatory in a "complete" cervical spine x-ray survey, a number of physicians, radiologists in particular, feel that two oblique views of the cervical spine are also necessary. We are of the opinion that the three-view cervical spine series is the minimum that should be obtained by the physician caring for all patients who are victims of multiple trauma. These views should be reviewed by the physician and with the radiologist as early as possible. If suspicion of injury exists, further radiologic studies may be obtained under the guidance, or with the assistance, of the radiologist or the orthopedic or neurologic surgeon.

Special studies that may be obtained include the oblique views men-

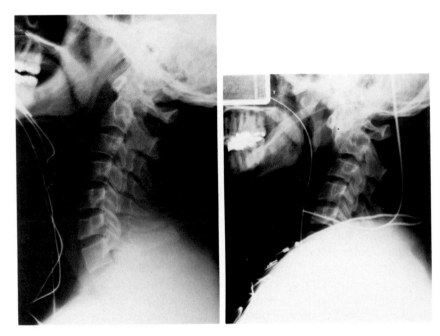

FIG. 4-2. Some fractures are not apparent when first x-rayed. Close evaluation of the initial films and follow-up films are important as this example, provided by Dr. Kimball Maull, demonstrates. The patient, although with a high alcohol level 0.40 vol %, had no neck pain, and a normal physical examination. (From Lieberman JF, Maull KI: Occult unstable cervical spine injury. *Journal of the Tennessee Medical Association*, April, pp. 243–244, 1988,. Used by permission.)

tioned previously, and if the lower cervical vertebrae cannot be visualized down to their articulation with the first thoracic vertebrae, a swimmer's view should be obtained. Similarly, if suspicion exists that a fracture may involve the articular pillar, then a pillar view should be ordered. Flexion-extension views in the lateral projection may be ordered, after appropriate consultation and under physician supervision, if a ligamentous injury resulting in an unstable cervical spine is suspected. Finally, the orthopedic or neurosurgery consultant may need further information about the location and extent of a cervical spine injury and obtain tomograms, CT scans, or three-dimensional CT views. All of these latter tests, however, fall into the province of the specialist consultant. Although it may be intellectually stimulating to achieve a precise anatomic diagnosis of the injured cervical spine, the vital function of the physician caring for the patient in the ED is to make the diagnosis that an abnormality is present and specialty consultation is required.

The physician treating the multiple-trauma patient must have some expertise at reading the three standard cervical spine roentgenograms. The first view reviewed is the cross-table lateral cervical x-ray, which may be obtained even in the resuscitation area using a portable x-ray machine. Physicians need to be aware that the roentgenogram with portable or fixed-target film equipment should be shot at a target-to-film distance of 100 cm (40 inches); however, the standard radiograph taken in the Radiology Suite is usually at a target-to-film distance of 6 feet, thus introducing a magnification factor of 2.5.[9]

It is suggested that because of the importance of the lateral film and the many details that can be extracted from it, the ED physician must have a standard plan, such as shown in Table 4-10, for reviewing this film. First, one should count vertebrae to ensure that all seven cervical vertebrae *and* their articulation with T_1 are seen (Fig. 4-3). Much data can be extracted even from such an inadequate film, but the view must be repeated until all vertebrae are seen (Fig. 4-4). The importance of this is obvious when remembering that C_7 is a common single site of cervical spine injury.[10] In some patients, particularly mesomorphic males, the lower cervical vertebrae may not be visualized, even with the use of gentle downward traction on the patient's arm. In this case, a "swimmer's" (Twining) view may be required. If adequate visualization is not obtained with this latter view, bilateral oblique views may need to be obtained.

The position or attitude of the spine should be noted. The normal configuration is a slightly lordotic curve, usually less in the supine or upright position. Any change to a flexed or kyphotic attitude, or rotation of only a portion of the cervical spine from the true lateral position, may suggest the presence of an injury.

TABLE 4-10.   **STANDARD PLAN FOR REVIEW OF CROSS-TABLE LATERAL CERVICAL RADIOGRAPH**

1. Count vertebrae
2. Check position
3. Assess for vertebral alignment
4. Inspect bony integrity
5. Measure spinal canal space
6. Examine intervertebral disc spaces
7. Review facet joints
8. Check spinous processes
9. Assess atlanto-occipital relationship
10. Inspect odontoid
11. Examine prevertebral soft tissues

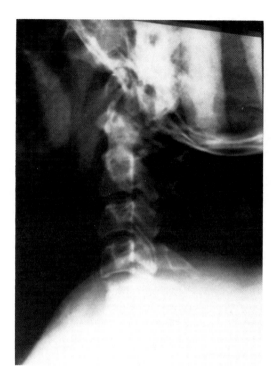

FIG. 4-3.   Inadequate cross-table lateral cervical radiograph.

The four lines of vertebral alignment should be inspected for irregularity. Normally, lines drawn down the anterior (anterior spinal line) and posterior (posterior spinal line) aspects of the vertebral bodies should be straight or gently curved. A similar line drawn through the posterior junction of the lamina, the spinolaminar line, should also be straight or regularly curved. Finally, a line placed through the tips of the spinous processes should also have a gentle and regular curve. Any irregularity of these lines may indicate the presence of a fracture or dislocation. Injuries resulting in disruption of these lines are often unstable because of ligamentous injury. Reference to the physiologic subluxation of C_2 to C_3 or C_3 to C_4 in children six years of age or less has already been made (Chapter 2).

The bony integrity of each vertebra should be examined. Note should be made of any disruption of the body, pedicles, lamina, or spinous processes. Though at times a difficult distinction to make, failure or incomplete ossification should not be mistaken for fractures, particularly in children.

The spinal canal (vertebral canal) space is measured from the pos-

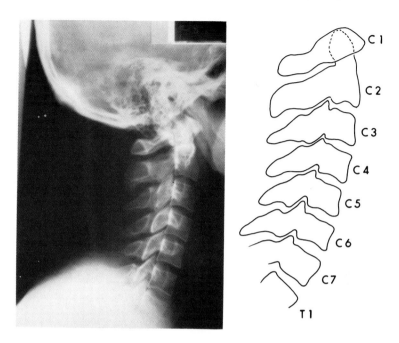

FIG. 4-4. Adequate cross-table lateral cervical radiograph (a) and illustration (b).

terior spinal line to the spinolaminar line. Because the spinal cord occupies 50% of the vertebral foramen below C_4 and one third of the foramen at C_1 to C_2, narrowing of this space beyond these limits may indicate spinal cord injury. At C_2 to C_3 the dura, pia, arachnoid and vessels reduce the clearance to only 1 mm anteriorly and posteriorly. In the normal adult, the minimal distance required to allow passage of the spinal cord and its associated parts is estimated to be 14 mm. A rough estimate may be made if the examining physician recalls that the width of the odontoid process is approximately the width of the cervical spinal cord.

Examination of the intervertebral disc spaces should show these to be similar in size at each level. Flexion injuries to the disc space may cause narrowing of the disc space, particularly anteriorly. Evidence that supports a traumatic cause for disc space narrowing is the presence of concomitant vertebral body compression fractures. Alternatively, hyperextension injuries will usually result in widening of the disc space, often at only one level. If the angle of inclination between adjacent vertebrae exceeds 11°, an unstable situation must be presumed to exist.[11]

The facet joints should show regular, smooth, and evenly spaced parallel joint surfaces. If the view is a true lateral, then the right and left facet joints should be superimposed. If the roentgenogram is not a true lateral, but is rotated, then all the facet joints on each side should have a similar degree of displacement. Any localized displacement of a facet joint is presumptive evidence of a subluxation or dislocation at that level.

The individual spinous processes upon examination should be intact, without evidence of fracture. In younger patients, secondary ossification centers at the tips of the spinous processes should not be mistaken for fractures. The space between the spinous processes should be regular. Any widening or narrowing of the interspinous space out of proportion to those above or below suggests injury.

Examination of the cervicocranium must be performed as well. This area is complex, but several normal anatomic features must be distinguished. First, the normal atlanto-occipital relationship should not be disturbed. The mastoid air cells, if developed, should project over the spinal cord and not over the vertebral bodies or spinous process. A line drawn along the clivus (located behind the sella turcica) should intersect the tip of the odontoid at the junction of the anterior and middle thirds of the odontoid.[6] Another line drawn tangential to the lamina of the atlas should intersect with the posterior foramen magnum.[12]

The odontoid process of the axis should be studied for evidence of fracture anywhere along its length. Care must again be taken in younger patients not to confuse incomplete or failed fusion of ossification centers with fracture. Similarly, at the tip of the odontoid, an os ossiculum should not be confused with a fracture. After the odontoid is studied for fracture, the atlanto-odontoid space should be measured. In adults, this should not exceed 3 mm and is usually only 2 mm.[13] In children, this distance may be up to 5 mm because of their greater ligamentous laxity.[13]

Finally, the soft tissues in the prevertebral space should be examined closely. At times, widening of this space may reflect edema and hemorrhage and may be the only indication of cervical spine injury. Unfortunately, prior placement of a nasogastric or endotracheal tube may distort this space and lessen the benefit of its measurement. Similarly, patient factors such as crying, swallowing, and performing a Valsalva maneuver may also effect the size of the space.[14] The prevertebral space may be divided into two components: a superior retropharyngeal space, and an inferior retrotracheal space. The normal width of the retropharyngeal space, measured in front of the body of C_2 or C_3, should not exceed 7 mm if performed with a 100-cm target-to-film distance; if standard technique is used with a 6-foot target-to-film distance, this space should be no wider than 4 mm.[9,14,15] If the target-to-film distance is unknown, a rough estimate of the upper limits of normal is 0.25% of the width (anterior-posterior) of the cervical vertebral body. In children, the retropharyngeal space should be no wider than two thirds the width of the second cervical vertebrae. In children, the retrotracheal space, measured at the anterior-interior margin of C_6, should not exceed 14 mm.[13] In adults, this space should be no more than 22 mm.[16]

The prevertebral space should also be studied for the presence of a prevertebral fat stripe. This stripe can be identified running along the anterior margin of the vertebral bodies to the level of C_6, where it deviates anteriorly over the scalene muscles.[17] It can be identified in most adults, but is seen less commonly in children.[6] Edema and hemorrhage from trauma to the anterior ligamentous complex, usually from hyperextension injuries, displace the fat stripe anteriorly.[17,18]

If repeated attempts to demonstrate the lower cervical vertebrae on lateral view fail, a swimmer's view should be obtained. The patient is positioned supine with the arm closest to the film extended cranially and abducted to 180°. This radiographic view is studied in a similar fashion to the lateral view, with particular attention being paid to the lower cervical vertebrae and cervical thoracic junction. The examiner must then make a mental summation of the lateral and swimmer's views and decide if abnormalities are present.

The open-mouth odontoid film (Fig. 4-5) is obtained with the patient supine and the x-ray beam centered over the open mouth and perpendicular to the film cassette. If overlying teeth or other obstructions to the x-ray beam obscure the odontoid, the beam may need to be redirected caudally or cranially to prevent overlapping of the shadows. Rarely, the Otanello technique, using a prolonged exposure time with the patient repeatedly opening and closing his mouth, may be useful to obtain an adequate film. The odontoid, lateral masses, and transverse masses of the altas should be particularly studied for evidence of fracture. Failure of ossification may result in parallel sclerotic lines about a radiolucent strip horizontally at the base of the odontoid, an os ossiculum, a bifid odontoid tip, or absence of a portion of the ring of C_1. In children, ossification of the neural arches, body, and odontoid is not usually complete until between the ages of three to six years. There should be no overhang of the lateral masses of the altas on the axis, and no disparity in the distance between the odontoid and either lateral mass. Finally, the bifid spinous process of the axis should be noted to be midline. If an adequate open-mouth odontoid view cannot be obtained, useful information can be gathered by review of a Towne's or reverse Water's view of the cranium.

An anterior-posterior cervical spine roentgenograph is taken with the patient again supine and the film cassette placed beneath the pa-

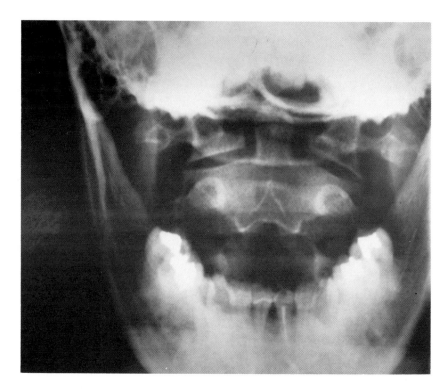

FIG. 4-5.   Normal open-mouth odontoid radiograph.

tient. The x-ray beam is angled slightly cranially and centered over the midcervical area. In this view (Fig. 4-6), the middle and lower cervical vertebrae are inspected for evidence of fracture in the body or transverse processes. The margins of the articular pillars should present a smooth, undulating line. The spinous processes should appear midline and equally spaced. Any change in one spinous process from midline is indicative of a unilateral locked facet.[6] A widening of any interspinous space of more than one-and-one-half times the interspinous space above or below correlates with the presence of a subluxation or dislocation.[19] If a double spinous process is seen, a spinous process fracture is likely present.[20]

Oblique views, if needed, are obtained with the patient again supine and the x-ray beam angled 45° from the midline, with a slight cephalad tilt, and centered over the midcervical region. The film cassette is placed behind the neck and angled so that the primary beam will impinge on it perpendicularly. Both right and left oblique views are obtained. These views are most helpful in studying the uncinate processes,

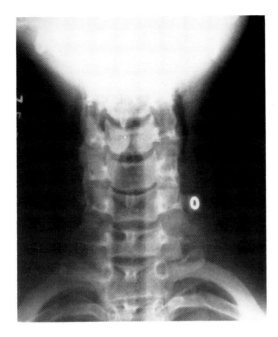

FIG. 4-6. Normal anterior-posterior cervical radiograph.

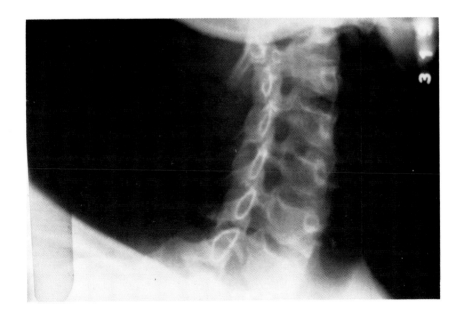

FIG. 4-7. Normal oblique cervical radiograph.

pedicles, laminae, and facet joints (Fig. 4-7). Facet joint subluxations or dislocations are particularly well seen.

A comprehensive approach to the initial assessment of the multiple-trauma patient with suspected cervical spine injury has been presented. The physician treating these patients should now have a concept of how to obtain a history, perform a physical examination, and order and interpret appropriate radiologic studies. Any abnormalities found in the clinical examination or radiographic evaluation of the patient mandate consultation with orthopedic or neurosurgical specialists.

REFERENCES

1. Committee on Trauma: *Advanced Trauma Life Support Course Instructor Manual.* Chicago, American College of Surgeons, 1985.
2. Maull KI, Sachatello CR: Avoiding a pitfall in resuscitation. The painless cervical fracture. *South Med J* 1977; 70:477–478.
3. Bresler MJ, Rich GH: Occult cervical spine fracture in an ambulatory patient. *Ann Emerg Med* 1982; 11:440–442.
4. Walter J, Doris PE, Shaffer MA: Clinical presentation of patients with acute cervical spine injury. *Ann Emerg Med* 1984; 13:512–515.
5. Medical Research Council: *Aids to the Examination of the Peripheral Nervous System. Memorandum No. 45.* London, Her Majesty's Stationery Office, 1976.
6. Berquist TH, Cabanela TH: The spine, in Berquist TH (ed): *Imaging of Orthopedic Trauma and Surgery.* Philadelphia, WB Saunders Company, 1986, pp 91–180.
7. Dunnington GL, Gervin AS: Cervical spine trauma: A review of 107 fractures in 90 patients. *J Trauma* 1983(A); 23(7):634.
8. Mace SE: Emergency evaluation of cervical spine injuries: CT versus plain radiographs. *Ann Emerg Med* 1985; 14:973–975.
9. Edeiken-Monroe B, Wagner LK, Harris JH Jr: Hyperextension dislocation of the cervical spine. *Am J Neuroradiol* 1986; 7:135–140.
10. Parks RE, Livoni JP: Detection of cervical spine injury in the multitrauma patient, in Blaisdell FW, Trunkey DD (eds): *Trauma Management, Cervicothoracic Trauma,* Vol. III. New York, Thieme, Inc., 1986, pp 56–65.
11. White AA, Johnson RM, Panjabimm P, et al: Biomechanical analysis of clinical stability in the cervical spine. *Clin Orthop* 1975; 109:85–96.
12. Christenson PC: Radiologic study of the normal spine. *Radiol Clin North Am* 1977; 15(2):133–154.
13. Locke GR, Gardner JI, Van Epps EF: Atlas-dens interval (ADI) in children. *Am J Roentgen* 1966; 97(1):135–140.
14. Martinez JA, Timberlake GA, Jones JC, et al: Factors affecting the cervical prevertebral space in the trauma patient. *Am J Emerg Med* 6:268–271, 1988.
15. Wholey MH, Bruwer AJ, Baker HL Jr: The lateral roentgenogram of the neck (with comments on the atlanto-odontoid-basion relationship). *Radiology* 1958; 71:350–356.

16. Weir DC: Roentgenographic signs of cervical injury. *Clin Orthop* 1975; 109:9–17.

17. Whalen JP, Woodruff CL: The cervical prevertebral fat stripe. *Am J Roentgenol* 1970; 109(3):445–451.

18. Forsyth HF: Extension injuries of the cervical spine. *J Bone Joint Surg* 1964; 46-A(8):1792–1797.

19. Naidich JB, Naidich TP, Garfein C, et al: The widened interspinous distance. A useful sign of anterior cervical dislocation in the supine frontal projection. *Radiology* 1977; 123:113–116.

20. Cancelmo JJ: Clay shoveler's fracture. A helpful diagnostic sign. *Am J Roentgenol* 1972; 115(3):540–543.

5

NORMAN E. MCSWAIN, JR.

Specific Fractures and Dislocations

INTRODUCTION

Injuries to the cervical spine can be classified as either fractures or dislocations (or a combination of fractures and dislocations). In turn, these injuries can be either stable or unstable. The dislocations can be partial or complete and locked facets can be associated with dislocations. An important consideration of such injuries is that the cervical spine can be fractured or dislocated, and even unstable, without producing neurologic damage. Only when impingement on the cord itself occurs by either the canal wall, a bony fragment, or the disc, does the neurologic function become compromised and the neurologic examination is abnormal. This can also be caused by ischemia or edema. Simply because the neurologic examination is normal, or as normal as can be detected (hampered by depressed level of consciousness from injury or overdose on alcohol or drugs), does not mean a fracture does not exist or that an unstable or potentially unstable situation is not present. The mechanism of injury must be used to heighten the examiner's index of suspicion so that immobilization is carried out until appropriate cervical spine films can be obtained to rule out fractures.

Stable Fractures

Usually, a fracture is stable if the bone is involved, but the supporting ligamentous structures have remained intact. In general, the three types of fractures are: compression fractures of the entire body (burst fracture), compression fractures of the anterior components of the body, and fractures of the processes (spinous and transverse).

Compression (Burst) Fractures

With this type of fracture, the entire body of the vertebra is compressed so that it is foreshortened both anteriorly and posteriorly, as well as laterally. The posterior elements are usually intact and the facets are not dislocated. Radiographically, the fracture can be identified by comparing the height of the vertebral bodies with those directly adjacent.

Anterior compression fractures can be identified by comparing the height of the vertebral bodies with those directly cephalad and caudad to the suspected injured vertebral body. Both the anterior and posterior components must be compared.

Process fractures break only those stabilizing and ligamentous attachment components of the spinous and transverse process. These usually do not affect enough of the supporting structures to be unstable.

Unstable Fractures

Unstable fractures, on the other hand, are ones in which a significant disruption occurs in the bony attachments of a supporting ligament or of the supporting ligaments themselves so that the stacked-block alignment of the vertebral bodies can no longer be maintained. The emergency physician must be most concerned with identifying such fractures so that external support of the vertebra can be maintained.

When a dislocation occurs and support of the "stacked blocks" is lost, impingement on the cord and neurologic damage result. In the area of C_3, the canal reaches its narrowest size in comparison to the cord contained within. There may be only 1 mm of clearance between the cord and its associated structures and canal wall at this point. Even minimal dislocation of the vertebral bodies can produce clinically significant compression on the vertebral cord with either resultant tearing of the nerve bundles or edema to produce ischemic injury. Partial dislocations can produce edema or the potentially unstable and overriding bones can compress the vertebral column. Adjacent disc space measurements identify significant unilateral or bilateral distraction of the involved vertebral bodies so that an unstable condition may exist.

Many possible combinations of these injuries exist. This text is not intended to identify the radiologic findings on all of those, or the subtle findings that may sometimes be seen. Rather, this text addresses the primary physician's identification of gross abnormalities and other possible abnormalities and their emergency management until more specialized care is available. For an in-depth discussion of these subtle findings, one is referred to the second edition of Radiology of Acute Cervical Spine Trauma by Harris and Edeiken-Monroe.[1]

STABLE FRACTURES

Compression (Burst) Fractures

Compression fractures occur as the entire force is delivered in a straight line along the anterior column compressing the body, rupturing the disc, or both, with occasional associated injury to the components of the posterior column. The supporting ligaments remain intact (see Fig. 2 and 6, Chapter 2). Bony components of the vertebral body, or extravasation of the intervertebral disc into the canal, however, can produce significant compression or penetrating injury of the spinal cord itself. Although these fractures can produce neurologic damage, they are usually stable.

Radiographically, the fracture is identified by significant shortening of the vertebral body both anteriorly and posteriorly, which may be associated with loss of intervertebral space distances. This fracture can be most readily identified by comparison of the intravertebral space as well as the body itself, with adjacent vertebral bodies in size and shape (Fig. 5-1).

Anterior Compression Fractures

Anterior compression fractures (Fig. 5-2) are distinguished from burst compression fractures in that the anterior-superior-inferior length of the vertebral body is less than the posterior-superior-inferior length. It is as if the vertebral body is wedged with the apex's wedge directed anteriorly and the base posteriorly. Although these are, in general, stable fractures, careful evaluation of the success to identify locking and the spinous processes to identify separation and tearing of the spinous ligaments is important radiologically. Neurologic damage may occur by the same mechanism as in the burst fracture described above. One also must be careful to distinguish this fracture from a teardrop fracture,

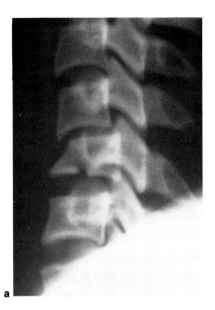
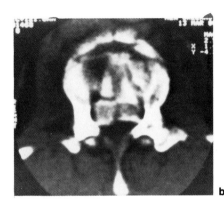

a
b

FIG. 5-1. (a) Compression fractures shorten the entire body of the vertebral body on all aspects; however, some components will compress more than others, producing an asymmetric profile. A compression fracture can be identified by comparing the shape and height of the vertebral body with the two bodies immediately cephalad and caudad to it. (b) Compression fracture frequently looks benign on plain X-ray. The computed tomography scan, however, shows an entirely different perception of the possible damages produced.

a hyperextension fracture with loss of anterior support of the cervical spine. The anterior wedge fracture may have lost posterior support.

If an anterior compression fracture is unstable, it will be unstable in the flexed position. Friends, relatives, and medical personnel who do not understand the severe consequences of this kind of injury tend to place pillows beneath the heads of patients with possible cervical spine injuries to provide comfort of the patient rather than being concerned with the medical consequences of their action.

Process Fracture

SPINOUS PROCESS
Fractures of the spinous process are most characterized by the so-called "clay shovelers fracture," which is an avulsion-type fracture of the spinous process of C_7 (Fig. 5-3). This can occasionally occur at C_6 and

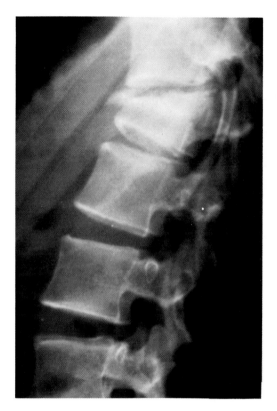

FIG. 5-2. Compression fractures resulting from flexion injuries frequently compress the anterior component of the body, leaving the posterior elements intact. The anterior wedging of this L$_1$ vertebra is a classic example of such changes.

T$_1$, but with less frequency. The "clay shovelers fracture" is a syndrome that developed in workers digging out clay with long-handle shovels. They had to throw the clay 12 to 15 feet out of the hole in which they were working. The shovel would stick in the clay, and force applied by the back muscles to move this mass out of its sticky environment would overcome the bony integrity of the lower cervical and upper thoracic spine, producing sudden pain and even an audible "pop." The modern fracture of the spinous process of the cervical spine is a forcible hyperflexion against tense paraspinal muscles. It is associated with automotive trauma or falls from heights. This fracture, which tends to be stable, is one of hyperflexion in trauma in which the spinous process ruptures, but not the spinous ligament.

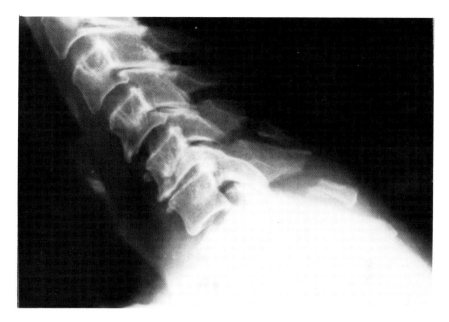

FIG. 5-3. Fractures of the spinous process such as the classic "clay shovelers fracture" can produce significant pain, but are stable. The distal portions of the spinous processes of C_6, C_7, and T_1 are broken off.

TRANSVERSE PROCESS

The transverse process is that portion of the vertebral body that extends out laterally attached to the trapezius or paraspinal muscles. A fracture of this component of the vertebral body does not impinge upon the cord and, therefore, is usually not one of major significance. It may have resulted from lateral flexion, however, and can to a limited extent represent a possible unstable neck fracture. Further down in the spinal column, these fractures are far less significant than in the cervical region, where the foramen for the vertebral artery can be involved and affect the cerebral blood supply. Awareness of this possibility must be a part of the primary physician's evaluation.

UNSTABLE FRACTURES

Jeffersonian Fracture (C_1)

The atlas or C_1 is significantly different from the rest of the cervical vertebra (see Chapter 2 and Fig. 2-2). Its body is, in actuality, the odontoid process. The support of the skull is on the interior-anterior surface of C_1 so that compression tends to force this ring laterally and apart. The result is usually a fracture of the ring in four places on either side of the anterior arches near the attachment of the structures to the facet (Fig. 5-4A).

In looking at a typical odontoid view, one can visualize the forces and their directions, translating this into expansion of the ring in the horizontal plane (Fig. 5-4B). An appreciation of the mechanisms and significance of this fracture can, thus, be gained.

The identification of this fracture is usually apparent on the odontoid view. Loss of symmetry occurs in relationship of the body of C_1 to the odontoid, as well as the facets between the skull and C_1 and C_2 (Fig. 5-5).

Fractures of the Odontoid

The normal anatomy of the odontoid is described in Chapter 2 (Fig. 2-3). Attention is called to the position of the odontoid inside the arch of C_1. In any other portion of the spine this would actually be the body of the cervical vertebra above. Embryologically, however, it develops

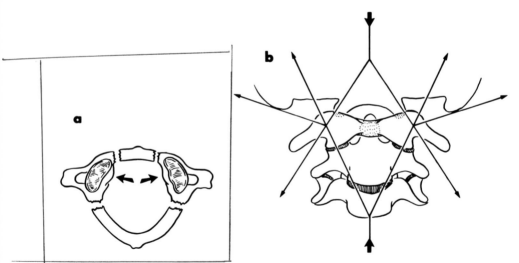

FIG. 5-4. (A) A Jeffersonian Fracture is a burst-type fracture of the ring of C_1. The more solid and larger component of the ring that has the facets are forced laterally. The ring then fractures in four places on either side of the anterior arch and where the posterior arches join the facets. (B) The anterior facets of C_1 articulate with the skull in such a manner that compression force on the skull pushes the facets laterally. As the force proceeds to C_2, the faceted area is again pushed laterally. This accounts for the type of fracture that occurs.

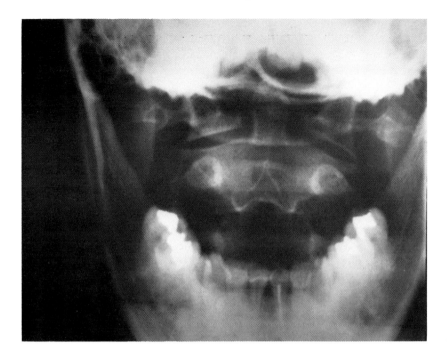

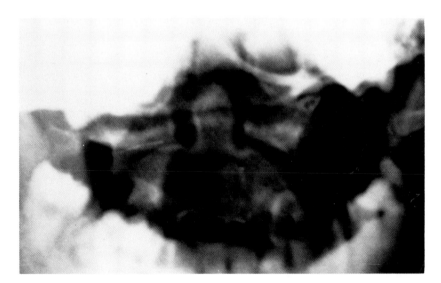

FIG. 5-5. Relationships between the odontoid and lateral masses should be equal. The spaces between the lateral masses and C_2 should be equal. The lateral border of C_1 should be aligned with the lateral border of C_2. Compare this roentgenograph with the one in Figure 5-7.

as a component of C_2 and by virtue of this embryologic development, we are able to turn our heads to look laterally in both directions. Maintaining the position of the odontoid and "its" relationship with C_1 is the anterior arch of C_1 and the transverse atlantal ligament (Fig. 2-4A and B). Preventing dislocation of C_1 from C_2 is the apical dental ligament running from the anterior part of the foramen magnum to the tip of the odontoid, the alae ligament, cunciform ligament. Other important supporting structures are between C_1 and C_2, which also have an important role in the odontoid C_1-C_2 stability.

In 1974 Anderson and D'Alonzo[2] described three types of fractures. Type 1 fracture (Fig. 5-6) involves the tip of the odontoid. This is probably an unstable fracture because it is similar to avulsion fractures of other bones in which the tendon is not disrupted but the tendon's attachment to the bone is pulled off. When a Type 1 fracture occurs, the possibility of loss of support of the apical dental ligament is paramount.

A Type 2 fracture occurs along the body of the dens, most commonly at its inferior portion where the dens fuses with the anterior arch and

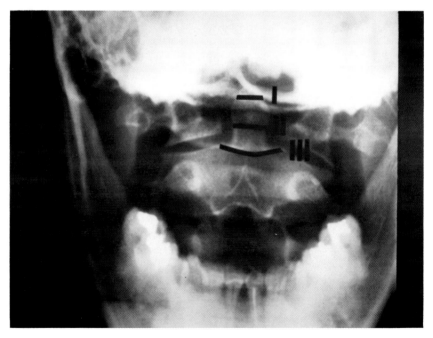

FIG. 5-6. Fractures of the odontoid can involve the tip (Type 1), the body (Type II), or the entire dens can be separated from C_2 (Type III). All are unstable because support provided by the apical dental ligament and transverse ligament is lost when the dens become detached from C_2 (see **Fig. 2-4A and B**).

body of C_2 (Fig. 5-6). This can also be an unstable fracture because the support of the transverse atlantal ligament has been lost.

A Type 3 fracture involves the body of C_1 and anterior arch. The os odontoideum has been described both as an ununited Type 2 fracture of the odontoid as well as an embryologic non-fusion of the odontoid to C_2. In the latter instance, this situation is stable; in the former incident it is probably unstable. When this situation (see Fig. 7-4A and B) is seen on the radiograph, it should be considered unstable until neurosurgical or orthopedic evaluations have determined otherwise.

Radiologic evaluation of the odontoid fracture of Types 1 and 2 is best visualized in the odontoid view (open-mouth) projection. Fractures along the body of the odontoid (Fig. 5-7) resulting in an unbalanced appearance of the relationship between the odontoid and C_1 or the relationship of C_1 to C_2, are clues to the presence of this fracture. Type 3 fractures can also be visualized in the odontoid (open-mouth) view.

The Mach effect is a regular lucent line extending across the body of the dens on the occipital view (Fig. 5-8). It is distinguished from a fracture because of its soft appearance as well as its extension beyond

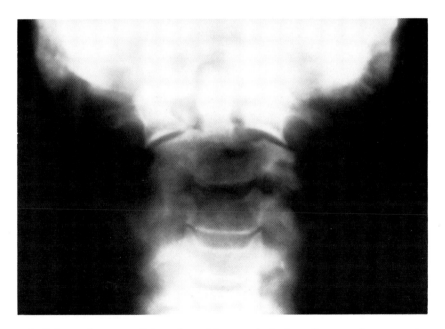

FIG. 5-7. A fracture of the odontoid not only looks off center, but may also allow enough instability of the C_1-C_2 relationship that it mimics and also may be combined with a Jeffersonian fracture. All such fractures are unstable. A computed tomography scan is necessary for exact delineation of the pathology.

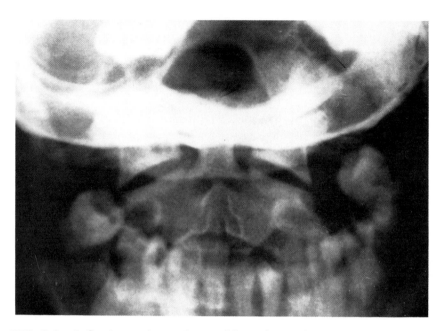

FIG. 5-8. Reflection and superimposed lines from other components of the skull and spine can produce a false impression of fractures. A classic example is the mock line overlying the base of the dens, which at first glance resembles a Type III fracture. Closer inspection, however, demonstrates that this line across the base of the dens proceeds laterally on each side. It can even be followed outside the confines of the neck and jaw on this view.

the odontoid across the disc space between C_1 and C_2 and out laterally beyond C_1. If this Mach effect cannot be identified as such and a question of a fracture exists, the odontoid view can be repeated in a slightly different projection to determine if the Mach effect moves, but the fracture line will not.

In the lateral radiographic view, the four major clues to the presence of an upper cervical fracture are: soft tissue swelling anterior to the vertebral bodies (Fig. 5-9); loss of relationship between the anterior arch of C_1 and the dens (maximum: 3 mm); visualization of a fracture line across the junction of the odontoid and C_2, which may be associated with a step-off (Fig. 5-10); or an extension of the fracture line down onto the body. The last sign is one of instability of the C_1-C_2 relationship and not specific visualization of the fracture. A straight line drawn between the posterior limits of the canal from C_1 to C_3 (Fig. 5-11) should be within 1 mm of the posterior canal limits of C_2. Posterior dislocation

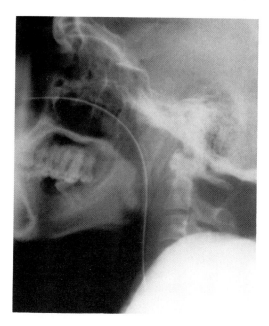

FIG. 5-9. The prevertebral space before the air contrast of the hypopharynx should be on 25% of the anterior posterior distance by the vertebral bodies in the area below C_3 or C_4. The esophagus begins and this relationship no longer applies.

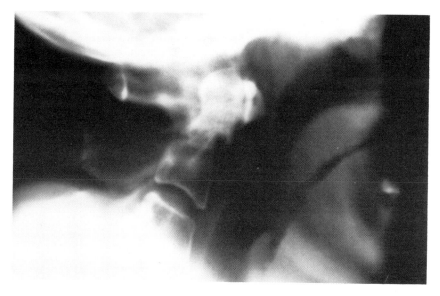

FIG. 5-10. A fracture of the odontoid may be difficult to see if not dislocated; however, if a definite step-off is present between C_1 and C_2 there is no question as to its presence. This is one of the four signs that should be checked each time an X-ray of the upper cervical vertebra is examined.

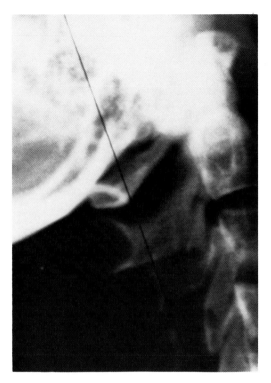

FIG. 5-11. A straight line drawn between the posterior canal line (anterior portion of the neural arch) between C_1 and C_3 should be within 1 mm of the posterior canal line of C_2. If this distance is greater, a fracture of the dens or C_2 should be suspected. The concern for instability and propensity for dislocation is real.

of C_2 beyond these limits should be an indication of instability between C_1 and C_2 and a possible fracture of the odontoid.

Hangman's Fracture (Traumatic Spondylolisthesis)

A hangman's fracture (whether intended as in capital punishment or from an accidental traumatic situation) produces a similar bony defect, although the kinematics of injury are different. In cases of capital punishment, a large knot is placed along the side of the head of the intended victim. As the trap door is released, the weight of the body is accelerated in a downward motion. The rope tightens laterally, flexing and rotating the head while the trunk continues its downward motion, which produces a fracture of C_2 and distraction of C_1 from C_2. In an accidental situation, neither the hyperextension nor hyperflexion is necessarily associated with distraction. The bony lesion is created at the pars interarticularis bilaterally, which is similar to the spondylolisthesis seen further caudad on the vertebral column characterized on the lateral view by a "collar" around the "Scotty dog's neck." Because an oblique view is not an available approach for this injury, the radiographic diagnosis has to be made on the more subtle findings of a fracture in the pars interarticularis, seen on the lateral stem of either one or both sides of the arch (Figs. 5-12 and 5-13). Enlargement of the ring is evidenced by > 1 mm posterior displacement of the posterior canal wall from the line drawn from the posterior walls of C_1 to C_3. An increase in the vertebral space between C_1 and C_2 may also be an indication of this fracture.

C_1 Neural Arch Fractures

Fractures of the C_1 neural arch are extremely subtle and unless close attention is given to this part of the anatomy, they will be missed.

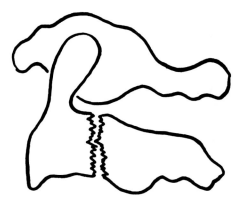

FIG. 5-12. This fracture through the pars interarticularis (Hangman's Fracture) can either be difficult to recognize or very obvious.

The fracture line usually extends downward with only a small amount of separation between the two bony fragments. Because one usually looks for a large spinous process as the most posterior component of the vertebral body, fractures of the C_1 neural arch can occasionally be confused with a spinous process fracture (Fig. 5-14). When one reviews the anatomy of C_1, however, it is clear that the spinous process of this neural arch is so small that a fracture is not a probability (Fig. 2-2).

Fractures C_3 to T_1

Fractures and dislocations of the C_3 to T_1 vertebrae are all similar in nature because the structure and ligamentous attachments are all

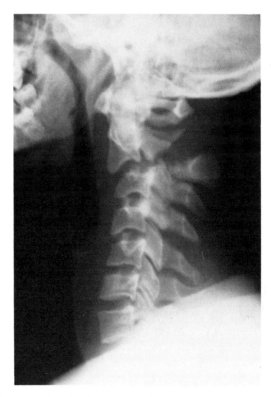

FIG. 5-13. The posterior displacement of the body of C_3 as related to C_2, loss of integrity of the pars interarticularis, posterior displacement of the posterior canal wall of C_2 as compared to C_1, and posterior position of the spinous process of C_2 make this Hangman's Fracture easy to recognize.

similar. Compression fractures and fractures of the spinous processes have been discussed above. This discussion is limited to fractures of the neural arch and fracture dislocations. The examiner must have a firm knowledge of the normal anatomy and the interrelationships between the various vertebrae, as discussed in Chapter 2. The fractures represent injuries to the posterior column, the supporting facet structure between the vertebrae. As discussed earlier, the anterior column is the body of the vertebra with its supporting intervertebral disc.

DISLOCATIONS

Dislocations are identified by malalignment of the vertebral bodies in one of the four lines of alignment. These are the lines along the anterior vertebral body that represent the anterior longitudinal ligament along the anterior portion of the canal—which essentially represents the posterior longitudinal ligament along the posterior border of the canal,

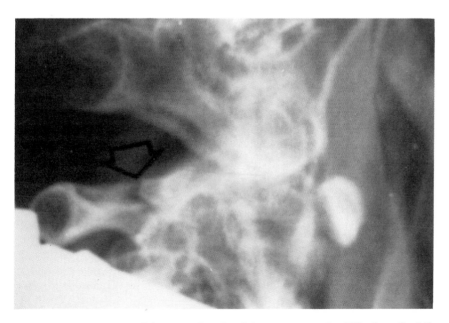

FIG. 5-14. Fractures of the neural arch of C_1 are extremely difficult to find if a specific close look is not taken each time a cervical spine roentgenograph is examined. The arrow and enlargement in this photograph of the radiograph make the fracture easy to find. Without these two factors on the original film this fracture is easily overlooked.

and finally, the projection of the most posterior aspects of the spinous processes (Fig. 5-15). Vertebral body malposition in any of these four areas should alert the examiner to a possible fracture or unstable condition in the involved vertebral body (Fig. 5-16). Close attention should then be directed along the neural arch and other aspects of the vertebral body for a small fracture line.

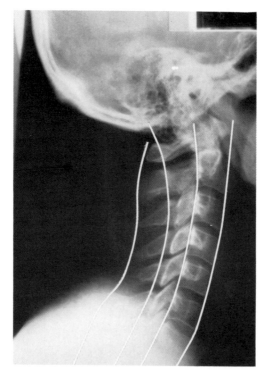

FIG. 5-15. Four lines should be smooth and flow from one vertebral body to another if the alignment is correct and no subluxations or dislocations are present. The first line touches the anterior part of the body of each vertebral body. The second line runs along the posterior line of the vertebral body. This represents the anterior border of the canal in which the cord lies. The posterior border of the canal is the anterior border of the neural arch. This is the third line that should be examined for alignment. The last alignment line is that which touches the distal (posterior) limits of the spinous process.

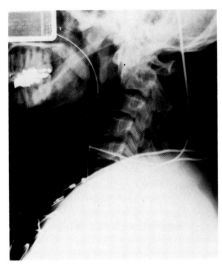

FIG. 5-16. When the vertebral bodies and canal walls do not align themselves, as described and depicted in Figure 5-15, a dislocation is present and the significant probability of compression of the cord by compromise of the canal lumen, as this picture from the case described by Dr. Kimball Maull from Chapter 4 presents.

REFERENCES

1. Harris JH Jr, Edeiken-Monroe B: *The Radiology of Acute Cervical Spine Trauma,* Ze. Baltimore, Williams and Wilkins, 1987.
2. Anderson LD, D'Alonzo RT: Fractures of the odontoid process of the axis. *J Bone Joint Surg* 54:1663–1699, 1974.

6

JORGE A. MARTINEZ

Cord Syndromes and Spinal Shock

COMPLETE AND INCOMPLETE CORD SYNDROMES

When the spinal column is involved in trauma, the spinal cord may be affected. The mechanisms of injury are flexion, extension, and axial loading, usually with a rotary component. This movement or rearrangement of the bones, ligaments, or discs can result in minimal to catastrophic injury to the spinal cord.

Areas of the spinal column most often injured are the cervical and lumbar spine; these two areas are prone to injury because of their mobility. They can be injured by direct force or indirectly by movements of the head or pelvis. The lower cervical region and thoracolumbar junction are the most common sites injured by indirect forces.[1] Craniospinal injuries also occur by direct and indirect forces. These lesions are extremely destructive with respiratory compromise, vasomotor paralysis, and rapid onset of death. This type of injury is rarely seen in the Emergency Department (ED).

The thoracic spine is more rigid and fixed because of the thoracic cage and, therefore, is rarely affected by blunt trauma. The spinal column is susceptible to penetrating trauma in all areas.

Injury to the spinal cord may be caused by direct physical transection (e.g., knife, bullet), vascular injury (e.g., anterior or posterior spinal artery injury), or edema or intramedullary bleeding with partial or complete physiologic transection. All of these mechanisms can cause damage ranging from transient functional loss to complete disruption of the cord with permanent paralysis.

Spinal concussion is also known as transient traumatic paralysis,[2] a diagnosis used to describe transient loss of some or most spinal cord function for only a few hours. Benes,[3] in his monograph, noted that complete loss of all cord functions is not seen in spinal concussion. In this situation, the spinal cord is intact, but edema or ischemia may cause disruption of function for a few hours. Recovery usually begins in six to eight hours, and complete recovery should return in 24 to 96 hours.

Contusion of the cord is more common and is caused by direct contact of the cord with displaced bone or soft tissues. The cord is usually intact, but is swollen or has a bluish discoloration. Microscopically, hemorrhage, tissue laceration, and necrosis are seen, especially in the gray matter. Rarely is the cord lesion confined to the area of injury, but rather can extend from one to several segments above or below the skeletal injury mainly because the skeletal segments and cord segments do not coincide (Fig. 6-1).[4]

Hardy and Rossier[4] reported that the limitations of anastomotic channels and effects of venous and arterial thrombosis have been found in progressive lesions that were thought to be caused by progressive spinal cord compression. Small thrombosed vessels can be found in almost all areas of medullary damage whether early or late. The spinal cord changes may start as small hemorrhages in the gray matter and progress to central necrosis with edema of the adjacent white matter and demyelinization. The entire segment(s) of the cord may eventually be involved. In cases of complete or incomplete lesions with return of neurologic functions, more severe edema usually occurs with less vascular involvement; therefore, as edema resolves, so does the neurologic involvement.

Finally, complete transection may occur via blunt or penetrating trauma. The transection or hemisection of the cord may be an actual physical disruption or a physiologic disruption. This may be caused by severe edema, intramedullary bleeding, thrombosis, hypoperfusion with ischemia, or a destruction of the spinal arteries to the section of the cord.

The presentation of spinal cord injuries is affected by the spinal shock syndrome. With an insult to the spinal cord, spinal shock ensues with the interruption of motor, sensory, and autonomic function at the level of the injury. Thus, spinal shock does not allow differentiation between a complete and incomplete lesion initially.

Complete lesions of the spinal cord result from anatomic or physi-

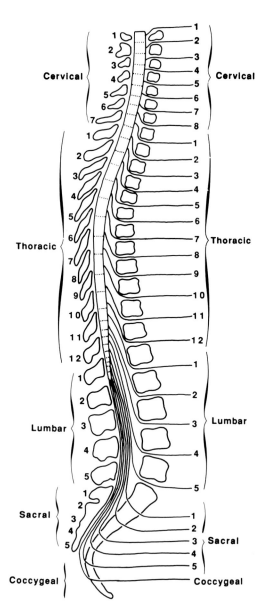

FIG. 6-1. Diagram illustrating the relationship of spinal column segments to spinal cord segments.

ologic transection of the cord. Sensory, motor, and autonomic function loss is bilateral and symmetrical. If motor or sensory asymmetry is found, or one or more reflexes are elicited below the level of injury, incomplete spinal cord injury becomes more likely. An example is "sacral sparing" in the presence of spinal shock, which implies that the anal wink and bulbocavernous reflexes are intact. This can alert the physician that, despite diffuse motor and sensory function defects, the sacral pathways are intact. The ascending and descending sacral tracts are on the peripheral aspect of the spinal cord; therefore, their preservation signifies that complete transection of the cord has not occurred (Fig. 6-2).

Complete spinal cord injury is combined with a slow resolution of spinal shock and persistence of symmetrical and bilateral paralysis, sensory loss, and autonomic dysfunction. This condition is followed by onset of spastic rigidity of the extremities below the lesion, persistence of sensory loss, autonomic dysfunction and lability, and the "mass reflex."

Incomplete lesions have preservation of motor and sensory function in an asymmetric or bilateral fashion. Another sign of an incomplete

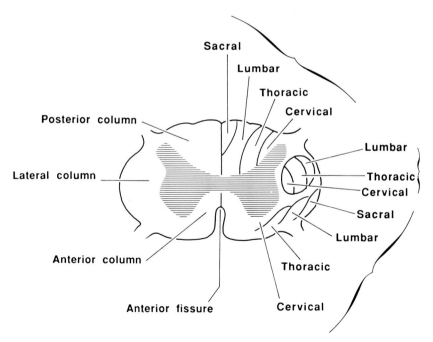

FIG. 6-2.   Illustration of spinal cord columns and alignment of cervical, thoracic, lumbar, and sacral tracts.

lesion is the return of functions previously absent below the level of injury. These facts reinforce the dictum that complete, detailed, and repeated neurologic examinations are essential in patients with spinal cord injuries.

Before describing the traditional incomplete syndromes, a brief review of the major anatomy of the spinal cord, cervical segment-muscle relationships, and sensory dermatomes is necessary. The spinal cord is composed of white matter, consisting of the ascending and descending motor and sensory tracts, and gray matter containing sensory and motor neurons. The dorsal horn is associated with sensory neurons; the ventral horn is associated with motor neurons.

The white matter is subdivided into three columns: dorsal, lateral, and anterior. The dorsal column contains the fasciculus gracilis and fasciculus cuneatus. These tracts are important for the sensations of proprioception, vibration, and touch. The fibers from the lower part of the body are more medially placed, and as the fibers enter the cord from higher up in the body, they are positioned more laterally.

The lateral column contains the lateral corticospinal tract among others. The corticospinal tracts (lateral and anterior) carry tracts for voluntary movement. They synapse with the motor neurons in the anterior horn of the gray matter. These fibers are placed laterally from the legs, and as one moves up the body, fibers in the tract are positioned medially.

The spinothalamic tracts are located in the anterolateral aspect of the lateral and anterior columns. They carry pain, temperature, and light touch. Most of these fibers desiccate in the white matter anterior to the central canal of the cord. These fibers are positioned similar to those of the corticospinal tract (Fig. 6-3).

Blood supply for the cervical spine is provided by the vertebral arteries, which eventually fuse to form the basilar artery. Before they join, however, each gives off a branch that fuses to form the single anterior artery, which runs in the ventral median fissure. This vessel supplies the anterior two thirds of the spinal cord and, therefore, supplies the ventral gray matter—anterior and lateral columns that include the corticospinal and spinothalamic tracts.

The posterior spinal arteries are paired and arise from the vertebral artery. These vessels supply the posterior third of the spinal cord, including the posterior columns and dorsal gray matter. It should be noted that anastomotic channels are not well established between the anterior and posterior spinal arteries.

Sensory dermatomes are demonstrated commonly by anatomic charts. Sensations to the back of the head and the neck are supplied by

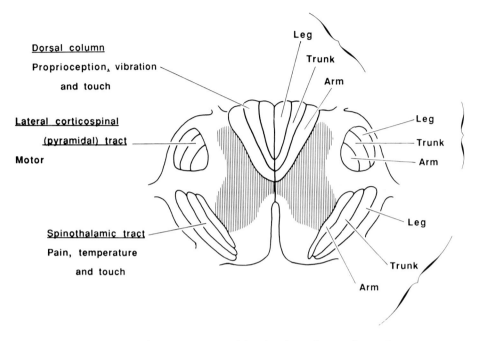

FIG. 6-3.   Diagram of major tracts and lamination of tracts by regions.

the C_2 and C_3 dermatomes; C_5 supplies the deltoid area; C_6 and C_7 supply the thumb; C_8 and T_1 innervate the little finger and anterior medial forearm; T_1 supplies the infraclavicular area; T_4 and T_5 supply the area of the nipple; T_{10} innervates the level of the umbilicus; and S_1 provides sensation to the little toe (Fig. 6-4).

Demarcation of dermatomes is not distinct and there is usually overlap of contiguous dermatome segments. Delineation of motor loss must be defined in cervical spine injury. Injuries of C_1 to C_3 cause respiratory depression because of their effect on the diaphragm and intercostal and abdominal muscles. Injuries at C_2 and C_3 will spare neck muscles (trapezius, sternocleidomastoid, and platysma) innervated by the spinal accessory and facial cranial nerves (cranial nerve VII). These may be the only muscles that can initiate inspiration and expiration.

Lesions at C_5 will cause paralysis of the deltoid, biceps, brachioradialis, and brachialis. Involvement at C_6 involves the triceps and extensor carpi radialis with concurrent weakness of the biceps, brachioradialis, deltoid, and brachialis.

Paralysis of the finger and wrist flexors and triceps muscles is seen

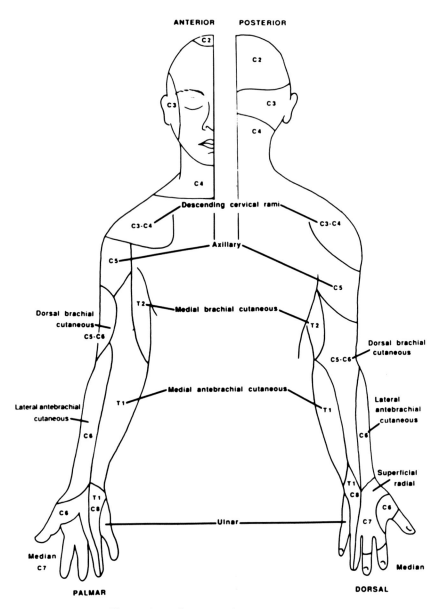

FIG. 6-4.   Gross illustration of sensory dermatomes.

with C_7 injuries. These patients will have good wrist extension, and the wrist will usually be extended at rest, because the extensor carpi radialis is innervated by C_6. Injuries at C_8 cause paralysis of the lumbricals and interossei, with a resulting claw hand. Lesions at T_1 cause motor loss of interossei, lumbricals, abductor pollicis, and abductor pollicis brevis, in addition to loss of all voluntary motion below the lesion. In all of these lesions, a loss of motor function occurs below the lesion, with weakness or decreased function in one or several spinal cord segments above the lesion because of the edematous and hemorrhagic changes in the spinal cord described previously.

Several well-described, incomplete cord lesions include the anterior cord syndrome, central cord syndrome, posterior cord syndrome, and Brown-Sequard syndrome. The physician should be aware of these syndromes; also, they may overlap or result in a variation of the classic syndrome. These incomplete syndromes have sparing of parts of the spinal cord, therefore, repeated neurologic examination will help delineate involved and uninvolved spinal cord functions. They also have a better prognosis in spinal cord trauma, with return of most or all neurologic function.

The anterior cord syndrome, caused by damage of the anterior horn cells and frequently the corticospinal tracts, was first described by Schneider in 1955.[5] The lower motor neuron involvement causes flaccid weakness and areflexia of all motor function below the level of the lesion. The posterior columns are preserved with retention of proprioception, two-point discrimination, vibration, and deep pressure sensation. It can be caused by flexion or extension forces, which can result in direct trauma to the cord by displaced bone or disc material, hypoperfusion with ischemia, or thrombosis of the anterior spinal artery that supplies the anterior two thirds of the cord.

A poor prognosis for recovery exists when the anterior cord syndrome is identified. Patients who have sparing of pain or temperature function, or retain even modest motor function below the level of the lesion, have a better chance of recovering at least some motor function. Reflex activity may return in the lower extremities, usually without the return of voluntary motor function.

The acute posterior cord syndrome is rare. In this syndrome, no loss of motor function or temperature is seen, but rather a loss of deep pressure, deep pain, vibratory sense, and proprioception. This type of injury often results from hyperextension, with involvement of the posterior elements of the spinal column causing direct damage to the cord or involvement of the posterior spinal arteries, with subsequent ischemia to the posterior column and gray matter of the cord. Patients often recover fully from this syndrome, but usually have ataxia to some degree.

The central cord syndrome is usually a result of hyperextension, especially in older patients with osteoarthritic changes of the spine. It is the most common type of incomplete spinal cord syndrome and is characterized by severe weakness or paralysis of the arms, and to a lesser degree, the legs. Bladder dysfunction, with urinary retention and abnormal control of defecation, may also occur. Sensory loss usually involves the pain and temperature tracts. The posterior column may also be involved with decreased or total loss of some or all of its functions. Horner's syndrome may be present if the ciliospinal center at C_8 and T_1 is involved.

Involvement of the upper extremities is usually a lower motor neuron flaccid paralysis, whereas involvement of the legs is a spastic upper motor neuron paresis or paralysis. The lesions are caused by hemorrhage and edema, which begin at the central canal of the cord and flare outward, and involve the gray matter predominately, with a varying degree of involvement of the white matter. When this occurs, the hemorrhage causes damage by compression of elements of the cord and, in some cases, repalcement of these elements with blood.

Better prognosis is seen in younger patients. Leg, bowel, and bladder functions usually return first. As the syndrome resolves, the ability to walk may return, but usually with some degree of spasticity. Arm strength then returns, followed by the hand proper, and then fine movements of the fingers. Complete return of fine-finger movements usually does not occur; therefore, the patient is left with residual motor defects in the upper extremities, especially in the hands and fingers.

The Brown-Sequard syndrome is usually the result of penetrating trauma from a bullet or knife, which causes a physical hemisection of the spinal cord. It results in: 1) ipsilateral upper and lower motor neuron defects, causing ipsilateral weakness or paralysis of the muscles below the lesion; 2) complete sensory loss at the dermatome level; 3) ipsilateral posterior column involvement, causing ipsilateral loss of position, vibration, and light touch; and 4) contralateral loss of pain and temperature sensations via involvement of the spinothalamic tract for several segments below the lesion. Bowel, bladder, and sexual dysfunction can occur, as well as hyperesthesia and vasomotor disturbances.

This syndrome is rarely seen in its pure, complete form and partial syndromes are more common. It may also be the result of blunt trauma. The syndrome generally presents with the motor damage greatest at the onset. Recovery is usually complete, although spastic paralysis of involved extremities may persist, as well as some degree of analgesia and thermoanesthesia.[6-11]

SPINAL SHOCK

"Spinal shock" has been observed as far back as Egyptian times, during the Pyramidal Age from 3000 to 2500 BC. Following is an account of this entity taken from the Edwin Smith Surgical Papyrus[12]:

> If thou examined a man having a dislocation in a vertebra of his neck, shouldst thou find him unconscious of his two arms (and) his two legs on account of it (and) while his phallus is erect on account of it, and urine drops from his member without his knowing it, his flesh has received wind, his two eyes are blood shot, it is a dislocation of a vertebra of his neck extending to his back bone which has caused him to be unconscious of his two arms (and) his two legs . . . an ailment not to be treated (p. 2).

"Spinal shock" is a term introduced by Marshall Hall in 1850, describing the transient suppression of nervous functions below the level of transection of the spinal cord. It is caused by interruption of ascending and descending fiber tracts (motor, sensory, and autonomic), with the temporary loss of all reflex activity, flaccid paralysis of the muscles and viscera, and loss of sensation below the injury.[13]

Sherrington and colleagues (cited in Guttman[14]) suggested that this transient depression of segments of the spinal cord below the transection is caused by sudden withdrawal of the predominately facilitating influence of descending supraspinal tracts from higher centers, resulting in a disruption of transmission at the synapses (including the presynaptic terminals, synaptic cleft, and subsynaptic membrane with its special receptive and reactive mechanisms). This disruption results in hypoactivity, flaccidity, and areflexia of the voluntary motor system. The interruption of sensory fibers leads to loss of all types of sensation below the injury. Autonomic involvement can lead to bladder paralysis, with urinary retention; ileus, with abdominal distension and constipation; and vasomotor involvement, with venous and arterial unresponsiveness causing hypotension, hypothermia, and reflex vagal bradycardia.

In a patient with spinal cord lesion, the initial presentation of spinal shock is hypotension. The hypotension is caused by loss of vasomotor tone, which causes increased venous capacitance with decreased venous return, as well as loss of arterial vasoconstriction with resulting vasodilation and decreased systemic vascular resistance. Bradycardia is also present because of interruption of sympathetic innervation of the heart and sparing of the vagal nerve with its parasympathetic innervation to the heart. This vagal predominance is seen commonly in lesions of T_4 and above. Other causes of hypotension and bradycardia that should be ruled out are inferior or anterior myocardial infarction with conduction system involvement, hypothyroidism, hypothermia, drug (barbiturate) or alcohol ingestion, and vasovagal reaction.

In the multiple-trauma patient, spinal shock may be superimposed on traumatic shock. The examining physician must give careful attention to the vital signs (hypotension with tachycardia versus bradycardia), in addition to gathering a detailed history including mechanism of injury, and performing a meticulous physical and neurologic examination. The neurologic examination should locate any neurologic defects. The physical examination should include location of chest, abdomen, or extremity trauma that may precipitate hypovolemia and evaluation of the spine for lesions that may precipitate spinal shock.

Treatment of shock in patients with pure spinal shock state is not accomplished with fluids alone. In this situation, the patient is not hypovolemic, but rather has lost the ability to control the vasculature. Resuscitation may require some fluid but the mainstay of therapy is the use of alpha-acting drugs to restore vasoconstriction and, therefore, systemic vascular resistance. Drugs used commonly include ephedrine, phenylephrine, and methoxamine. Indiscriminate volume resuscitation may cause fluid overloading, with signs and symptoms of volume overload, when vascular regulation returns.

In cases of combined hypovolemic and spinal shock, fluid resuscitation is required, but an awareness of a concurrent vasomotor dysfunction is essential. Fluids and blood products, therefore, should be used to correct hypovolemia, but these should be monitored carefully along with blood pressure response and urine output (via urinary bladder catheterization). The patient must also be monitored for several days for signs and symptoms of volume overload, such as hypertension, cardiac failure, pulmonary congestion, peripheral edema, or excessive urinary output.

Management of hypotension is important because of conjecture that the shock state with its hypotension and resultant hypoperfusion may worsen damage sustained in cord injury by worsening ischemia.

The respiratory depression that occurs in spinal shock can also be devastating and must be addressed initially. Injuries to the cervical cord can cause loss of the diaphragm (C_3, C_4, C_5), intercostal muscles (thoracic cord), and abdominal muscles (thoracic and lumbar cord) and can cause severe depression of respiratory function. Airway protection and ventilation control are necessary while the shock state is being addressed.

Spinal shock can last for variable periods of time, from days to weeks in severe injuries or from minutes to hours with slighter injuries. It may also be difficult to evaluate the extent of spinal cord damage because this syndrome may be present in complete and incomplete spinal cord injuries.

Because of the length and complexity of the spinal shock syndrome, organ system involvement may occur that can be detrimental to the patient, acutely and in the long term. The respiratory system is almost invariably involved in cervical spine injuries. If the lesion occurs above C_3, the phrenic nerve to the diaphragm and intercostal and abdominal muscle function will be lost. This condition will cause decreased total capacity and tidal volume with resultant hypoventilation. Respiratory support in this situation is mandatory.

The trapezius and sternocleidomastoid muscles are also used in respiration and are supplied by the spinal accessory nerve (cranial nerve XI). These are not involved in high cervical spine injuries. Lesions that spare the diaphragm allow better ventilation spontaneously, but the loss of thoracic and abdominal muscle function hinders the ability to maximize inspiratory and expiratory phases and clear the lungs of secretions. Complications may occur later because of the inability to cough and clear secretions. This may lead to respiratory obstruction, atelectasis, and pneumonia.

Function of the urinary bladder is involved in spinal shock. Voluntary and reflex voiding is inhibited by paralysis of the detrusor, striated bladder, and urethral muscles. The external and internal sphincters remain closed. The bladder, therefore, distends with a gradual increase in intravesicular pressure that eventually overcomes the sphincter muscles causing escape of droplets of urine (overflow incontinence). This distension can result in bladder atony if regular bladder emptying is not instituted. Management consists of a closed-system indwelling catheter initially, which is replaced with intermittent catheterization as the spinal shock resolves. This helps prevent urinary tract infection by decreasing bladder volume and ridding of residual volume, which can be used by bacteria as a culture medium for growth. It also helps to maintain the muscle tone of the intrinsic bladder muscles for reestablishment of reflex bladder activity. This maintenance of bladder function helps prevent excessive intravesicular bladder pressure, which can cause hydronephrosis and precipitate renal failure. Calcium stone formation may occur secondary to high calcium turnover from bone resorption due to immobilization of the patient. Adequate kidney and bladder function can help decrease the incidence of these stones.

The gastrointestinal system develops acute atony of the stomach and small and large intestines. Ileus with abdominal distension may occur. Gastric atony with resulting distension can cause vomiting with pulmonary aspiration along with decreased diaphragmatic motion. The patient may develop constipation, fecal impaction, or both, because of colonic atony and loss of reflexes controlling defecation. Fecal incontinence may develop secondary to decreased or lost sphincter tone. Gastroduodenal hemorrhage may develop because of stress ulceration, which can progress to perforation with peritonitis.

Gastrointestinal problems may be alleviated with nasogastric intubation for the gastric distension, antacids or H^2 histamine receptor blockers for gastric ulceration, and use of laxatives or stool softeners to control bowel problems. The nasogastric tube should be left in place until gastric atony resolves. The patient should not be fed enterally until the atony resolves.

Vascular stasis, because of the pooling of blood in the venous system, will lead to deep vein thrombosis in almost all patients. These may eventually embolize, especially if motion returns or if the patient is moved. Whenever possible, prophylactic anticoagulants should be started, being mindful of the effect they may have on gastrointestinal bleeding. Antiembolic stockings should be applied early in patient care. The dependent immobile extremities may develop edema because of the stasis of blood.

As stated previously, vasodilatation occurs because of loss of sympathetic control—the so-called functional sympathectomy; therefore, hypotension resulting from increased venous capacitance and decreased vasoconstrictor control occur. Swelling of soft tissue and flushing of skin occur because of this vasodilatation. Nasopharyngeal mucosa may swell with resultant blockage of the nasal air passage (Guttman's sign), causing difficulty in breathing and swallowing. It is important to remember that there will be no vascular response to change in positions during the temporary vasomotor paralysis. If the patient's position is changed in a vertical plane, therefore, there will be immediate and uncontrolled orthostatic hypotension.

Horner's syndrome may also be present because of interruption of the oculopupillary fibers that originate in the hypothalamus and descend in the anterolateral tract, which is in the intermediolateral horns of C_8 to T_2. The patient will have miosis (because of paralysis of the dilators of the pupil), flush of face and nasal congestion (because of vasoconstrictor loss), loss of sweating (because of sympathetic disruption), and ptosis of the eyelids. This occurs most commonly with cervical spine injuries.

Spinal shock may also include problems with temperature regulation because vasodilation allows heat loss, inability to shiver prevents heat conduction, and loss of sweat gland function prevents temperature regulation. The skin may, therefore, be warm, flushed, and dry.

With the loss of vasomotor and sphincter control, erection of the penis may occur with transection of the cord. Patients with this phenomenon and a history of trauma should bring spinal cord injury to mind immediately. This phenomenon is transient; however, development of priapism is an ominous sign of severe and usually complete cord transection, especially if it lasts more than several hours.

Spinal shock is not a permanent state; it may last from several hours to months. As function returns, it usually does so from a caudal to cephalic route. The reflexes that appear first are the anal and bulbocavernous reflexes and reflexes to plantar stimulation. Paralysis below the lesion will remain, but becomes spastic rather than flaccid because of the loss of higher cortical inhibitory control of spinal reflex arc. Movement is a withdrawal from any stimulus, therefore, because of the lack of modification or control by the higher cortical centers. These cortical centers modify spinal reflex arcs and prevent exaggeration during an appropriate response to the stimulus.

With loss of these centers, all stimuli, whether normal or threatening, precipitate the same exaggerated responses. This phenomenon is called the "mass reflex," where sensory stimuli may cause nonpurposeful violent withdrawal movements of the extremities below the lesion along with induction of profuse sweating and bladder and rectal emptying. These, too, are a result of exaggerated uncontrolled reflex arcs (voluntary and autonomic) below the level of the spinal cord lesion.

As the spinal shock syndrome regresses, the autonomic function of the bladder and bowel returns to normal with reflex autonomic evacuation secondary to stretch of the organ. This emptying, however, may be triggered by an unrelated stimulus, such as rubbing the foot or scratching the abdomen. Another sequela of cord transection is that patients with these lesions remain sensitive to catecholamines (endogenous or exogenous) for the rest of their lives. In these situations, medications may be necessary to control the unwanted, indiscriminate, autonomic function that can result from "extra-autonomic" stimuli.[6,8,9,15,16]

REFERENCES

1. Jellinger K: Neuropathy of cord injuries, in Vinken PJ, Bruyn GW (eds): *Handbook of Clinical Neurology,* Vol. 25. Amsterdam, North Holland Publishing Company, Amsterdam, 1976, pp 43–122.

2. Black P: Injuries of the spine and spinal cord: Management in the acute phase, in Zuidemia GD, Rutherford RB, Ballinger WF, Black P (eds): *The Management of Trauma,* ed 3. Philadelphia, WB Saunders Company, 1979, pp 226–253.

3. Benes V: *Spinal Cord Injury,* London, Balliere, Tendall, and Cassell, 1968.

4. Hardy AG, Rossier AB: *Spinal Cord Injuries: Orthopedic and Neurologic Aspects,* Germany, Thieme Publishing Sciences Group, Inc., 1975, pp 1–97.

5. Schneider RC: The syndrome of acute anterior spinal cord injury. *J Neurosurg* 1955;12:95.

6. Yashon D: *Spinal injury,* New York, Appleton-Century-Crofts, 1978.

7. McQueen JD, Khan MI: Evaluation of patients with cervical spine injuries, in Cervical Spine Research Society (eds): *The Cervical Spine.* Philadelphia, JB Lippincott Co, 1983, pp 128–140.

8. Weiner SL, Barrett J (eds): *Traumatic Management for Civilian and Military Physicians,* Philadelphia, WB Saunders Company, 1986, pp 122–126.

9. McSweeny T: Fractures, fracture dislocations, and dislocations of the cervical spine, in Jefferies E (ed): *Disorders of the Cervical Spine.* London, Butterworths, 1980, pp 48–79.

10. Green BA, Magana IA: Spinal cord trauma, in Davidoff RA (ed): *Handbook of the Spinal Cord,* Vols. 4,5. New York, Marcel Dekker, Inc., 1987, pp 63–96.

11. Braakman R, Denning L: Injuries of the cervical spine, in Vinken PJ, Bruyn GW (eds): *Handbook of Clinical Neurology,* Vol. 25. Amsterdam, North Holland Publishing Company, 1976, pp 227–380.

12. Bennet G: History, in Howorth MB, Petrie JB, Bennet G (eds): *Injuries of the Spine,* Baltimore, Williams and Wilkins Co., 1964, pp 1–59.

13. Howorth MB, Petrie JG, Bennet G: Neurologic injury. *Injuries of the Spine.* Baltimore, Williams and Wilkins Co., 1964, pp 276–333.

14. Guttman L: Spinal shock, in Vinken PJ, Bruyn GW (eds): *Handbook of Clinical Neurology,* Vol. 26. Amsterdam, North Holland Publishing Company, 1976, pp 243–262.

15. Tator CH, Rowed DW: Current concepts in the immediate management of acute spinal cord injuries. *CMA J* 1979;1453–1464.

16. Soderstrom CA, Brumback RJ: Early care of the patient with cervical spine injury. *Orthop Clin North Am* 1986;17(1):3–13.

7

JORGE A. MARTINEZ

Cervical Spine Injuries in Children

One of the most devastating and anxiety-provoking situations in the Emergency Department (ED) is the child with a potential cervical spine injury. Luckily, this is not a common occurrence, but because of the potential morbidity and mortality, it is a situation that requires an intelligent and organized evaluation. It also requires a basic understanding of the common skeletal variations that can be seen in the child. The fundamental, basic evaluation of the traumatized child is also necessary. In this section, the precipitating environmental factors, skeletal variations, evaluation, and presentation of the child with cervical spine injury are discussed.

Most injuries involving the cervical spine in the child or adolescent are caused by motor vehicle accidents and sports-related injuries—mainly swimming and diving accidents. Boys are involved twice as often as girls. A combined study, including the California epidemiologic study (58 children) and the Institute for Rehabilitation and Research in Houston (97 children), was done to find common causes of cervical spine injury. Fifty-two percent of the spinal injuries were from motor vehicle collisions (80 children). Of these 80 children, 57% were passengers in an automobile or pick-up truck, 26% were pedestrians, 9% were bicyclists, and 7% were on motorcycles. Twenty-seven percent of the injuries were sports-related, such as diving, football, wrestling, boxing, or horseback riding. Accidental firearm injuries accounted for 13% of the 155 cases. Falls accounted for 6% of the total cases. One of the 155 children, a two-year-old, had cervical spine injuries secondary to child abuse.[1]

Caffey[2] in 1974 and Swischuck[3] in 1969 described a form of child abuse, called "whiplash shaken infantile syndrome," caused by the child being shaken violently. Violent shaking causes the large head of the child to be moved back and forth over the weak neck muscles, resulting in intracranial and intraocular hemorrhages that cause neurologic and visual defects. Spinal column and spinal cord injuries have also been reported.

Cervical spine injuries are associated commonly with head injuries, especially as a result of direct trauma to the head with transmission of the forces to the neck. All head injuries, therefore, must have cervical spine injuries ruled out clinically and radiologically. It is often difficult, however, to do an organized, meaningful neurologic examination in small children and infants. In this situation, the child must be observed for spontaneous movements, because "mass reflex" movements to stimuli (uninhibited spinal cord reflexes in response to a stimulus) may give the impression that normal movements are intact.

A clue to help distinguish voluntary movements from spinal cord reflexes is that if a painful stimuli is given above the level of cord injury, there will be no movement of the limbs affected by the injury. If the stimulus is given below the cord lesion sensory level, however, a reflex withdrawal will occur, but will not produce an irritable response by the child. Also important is an irritable response (such as crying) by the child to a painful stimulus above the cord lesion, whereas there will be no such response to the stimulus if applied below this lesion. Lack of sweating with flushed skin or respiratory difficulty (caused by involvement of the diaphragm, intercostals, and abdominal muscles) may also indicate a spinal cord lesion. Obviously, repeated neurologic examination and observation is imperative for discerning these signs of injury.

When a child is brought to the ED with a suspected cervical spine injury, the spine should be immobilized immediately, if it was not done previously in the field. This is rarely a problem today, because national teaching programs with certification of Emergency Medical Technicians include proper prehospital evaluation and patient transfer techniques for emergency care. It is clearly inappropriate for a victim of any trauma with a chance of spinal injury to be transported without proper immobilization; however, should this have occurred, prompt immobilization should be done. This may help prevent an uninjured or partially injured cord from sustaining more damage.

After or during the immobilization, airway management with an intravenous (IV) access (two peripheral IVs—optimum) should be started. Primary survey of airway, breathing, circulation, and neurologic status is also performed initially. Management of life-threatening injuries with aggressive resuscitation of hypovolemia and hypotension is critical. This can help prevent or manage the shock state. There is speculation that hypotension may aggravate spinal cord injuries by causing sustained hypoperfusion of the spinal cord with resulting ischemia and infarction.[4]

Tracheal intubation may be needed to protect the airway or ventilate the patient. If indicated, the procedure should be done with the head and neck in a neutral position. Traction may cause further damage to the cord because distraction of the vertebra can occur in unstable fractures. Either nasotracheal or endotracheal intubation can be undertaken using the route that will be best tolerated and cause the least amount of movement and trauma. Surgical cricothyroidotomies should not be done in young children because accidental incision of the cricoid cartilage may allow the trachea to collapse, thereby closing the airway. When the airway has been cared for and resuscitation started, a complete secondary survey with neurologic examination should be performed. This should be repeated while the patient is in the ED and as disposition and consultations are prioritized.

When the child's vital signs are stabilized, or if immediate surgical intervention is needed, a lateral cervical spine radiograph should be obtained. It is imperative that all seven cervical vertebrae are seen. The films should then be studied extensively for signs of trauma, remembering that anatomic variations may make this difficult.

Burke,[5] in 1974, reported that 50% of children with major neurologic involvement had normal roentgenograms. Kewalramani,[1] in his review, reported that 47 of 196 children aged one to 18 years with spinal cord injuries had radiologic studies without any abnormalities, but 119 had definite evidence of injury on plain radiographs.

The reason accepted most commonly for the high incidence of normal radiographs with associated neurologic deficit is that the vertebral column in children is extremely elastic, more so than the spinal cord. This is because of the laxity and strength of the ligaments of the vertebral column, ability of the discs to stretch, and an inherent flexibility of the spine that allows the spinal column to move in more extreme directions (flexion, extension, lateral movement) without damage. The spinal cord, however, is relatively fixed in place by the dentate ligaments, spinal nerve roots, and blood vessels.

In hyperflexion, the spinal column can bend further than the spinal cord and its dura can stretch. The dura may tear, therefore, and the spinal cord itself may tear apart completely or be stretched severely by longitudinal traction resulting in edema and intramedullary hemorrhage into the cord. There may also be damage to the associated vascular structures with hypoperfusion or thrombosis that can cause further ischemia and damage.

In hyperextension, the spinal column can become compressed to the point of extraction of vertebral elements. The spinal cord, again being less elastic, may become compressed like an accordion, which can precipitate edematous, hemorrhagic, and vascular changes. The extreme movement of the vertebra may squeeze the cord between the lamina and vertebral body and cause damage. Distracted vertebrae may directly traumatize the cord and then undergo subsequent spontaneous autoreduction, leaving little or no gross evidence of cord damage. Autopsy findings of children sustaining these types of injuries have shown prevertebral hemorrhage, edema, hematomyelia, and cord infarction.

It is important to remember that radiographs are a view of a static situation and may not demonstrate the injury that occurred with the spine in a different position. The hypermobility of the cord, therefore, may actually allow an injury to occur in a dynamic situation that may be difficult to identify in a static state.

The hypermobility of the spinal column that can produce angles and translocations, which appear abnormal, combined with a variety of ossification centers can cause the immature spine to mimic traumatic lesions on x-ray. Common variations involve the C_2 to C_3 and C_3 to C_4 levels and the atlas and axis, especially the odontoid.

In the child, ossification centers are usually fused completely by 12 years of age. As a result, these ossification centers may mimic fractures (Figs. 7-1, 7-2, and 7-3).

The lateral masses of the atlas are ossified at birth. The posterior arch of the atlas develops by extension from the lateral masses, thereby closing the arch at about three years of age. The atlantal anterior arch develops an ossification center at about one year of age and fuses with the lateral masses by the sixth to ninth year of age.

The odontoid has an ossification center that may be bipartite at birth. At two years of age, an apical epiphysis appears and fuses with the main body of the odontoid by age 12. The main odontoid body then fuses with the body of the atlas at four to seven years of age. Occasionally, the junction of these two bodies may retain a subdental cartilaginous tissue called the subdental synchondrosis or os ondontoideum, present in about 4% of children.[6] This variation is important because the nonossified area can be confused with a fracture at the base of the odontoid.

The ossification of C_3 to C_7 occurs similarly. At birth, each vertebra has a paired center for each half of the vertebral body itself. The arch

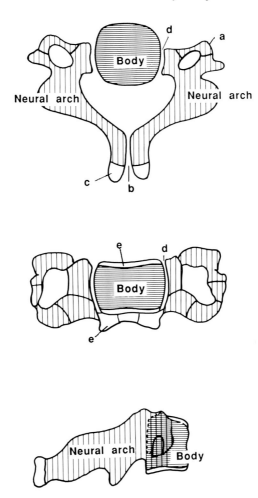

FIG. 7-1. First cervical vertebra: (a) body ossification begins to appear by one year; (b) neural arches ossify in utero, and the spinous processes (c) have united by 32 to 40 months. The arch unites with the body (d) between the sixth and eighth years, whereas the vertebral notch remains a ligament for many years.

ossification centers extend into the vertebral bodies and produce a neurocentral synchrondosis that may be apparent in the spine until fusion occurs at three to six years of age. The vertebral arch closes at two to four years. Secondary ossification centers may persist at the tips of the transverse and spinous processes.

Synchondrosis of ossification centers must be differentiated from fractures, but this may be difficult. Fractures are usually irregular, congruent, and rarely in the areas of ossification centers. Synchondroses

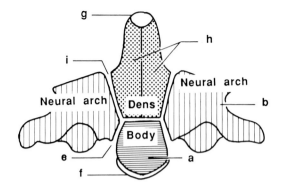

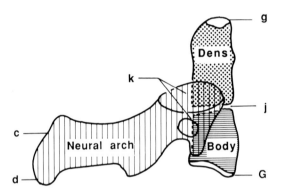

FIG. 7-2. Second cervical vertebra: (a) the body develops earlier than the C_1 body. It begins to ossify in utero (5 mo). The neural arches (b) ossify in utero also, one or two months after the body and are fused (c) at 30 to 36 months. The tip (d) is usually split. The arches fuse to the body (e) during the latter part of the first five years of life. The inferior epiphyseal ring (f) is fused in the first quarter century of life. It may be visible as early as ten years. The center at the top of the odontoid is visible by five to six years of age and solid by age 12 (g). The dens develops (h) as two parts but fuses in utero. The odontoid and neural arch (i) are fused by six years, as are the body and odontoid (j).

appear as smooth areas with sharp borders and are darker and more distinct on x-ray than fracture lines.

The C_2 or C_3 psuedosubluxation is a common variation that can mimic fracture on a child's cervical spine film. Cattell and Filtzer[7] reported a 24% incidence of this finding in children one to seven years old. Reasons stated for this variation were: 1) extreme mobility of the cervical spine of children; 2) fulcrum for cervical movement at

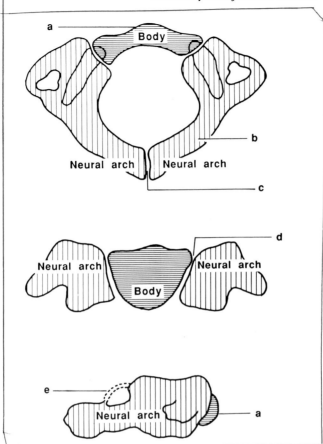

FIG. 7-3. From C_3 to C_7 the vertebrae look similar and the ossification centers fuse at the same time. The anterior portion of the neural arch has joined the main component by age six. The arches fuse (b) by two to three years of age, and the secondary centers (c) are visible at puberty but do not fuse until about age 25. The body and arches (d) fuse at about the same time as this area on C_1 and C_2. The fusion is complete by age 6. The superior and inferior rings do not completely fuse for the first 25 years.

C_2; and 3) relatively horizontal position of the C_2 to C_3 articular facets, allowing the anterior movement. Sullivan, Bruwer, and Harris,[8] in 1958, described up to 4.0 mm anterior subluxation of C_2 on C_3 and C_3 on C_4,[9] which is also related to the ligamentous laxity of the vertebral column, especially at these levels.

In mild flexion of the child's cervical spine, a slight amount of step-off is usually present; however, with exaggerated forward flexion, step-offs may occur with up to 3 to 4 mm anterior displacement over the subjacent vertebra.[7] Children also tend to have an absence of cervical lordosis and flexion curves. Soft tissue changes can occur without skeletal injury. This is especially true in children who are screaming, because screaming or exhalation may cause the prevertebral space to widen. This can be corrected by taking the radiograph with the child relaxed and during inspiration.

The immature spine has anterior wedging of the vertebral body, which may be misinterpreted as a compression or chip fracture by the unwary physician. Ossification centers of the transverse and spinous processes or apical ossification center of the odontoid process may be interpreted incorrectly as avulsion fractures.

The atlas moves easily anteriorly and posteriorly because of ligamentous laxity. In extension, the atlas appears to slide up over the distal end of the odontoid; as much as two thirds of the anterior arch can be above the ossified odontoid. This occurs because the tip of the odontoid is unossified, and the atlas moves distally over the ossified odontoid to the level of the distal unossified odontoid. Cattell and Filtzer[7] documented that this occurred in 20% of normal children. With flexion in a child, the interval between the atlas and odontoid can be as much as 4 to 5 mm. This interval is usually not greater than 3 mm in adults.

The odontoid process has several ossification centers, one at the base of the vertebral body, one at the distal odontoid, and sometimes in the midline. These ossification centers should be kept in mind when interpreting films. Lastly, the function of the odontoid fuses with the body of the axis at seven or eight years of age, which may be confused with a fracture before fusion. When fusion occurs, however, there may be a thin cartilaginous line that remains to mimic a fracture—the os odontoideum (Fig. 7-4).

After evaluating the films for normal variations, a search for real fracture can be undertaken. Several types of fractures are common in children. The most common fractures are to the odontoid, atlas, axis, and C_2 to C_3 area. Injuries below the third cervical vertebra in children are so rare that significant data have not been accumulated.[10]

In one reported series,[11] lesions of the atlas and axis occurred in 16% of adults but in as much as 70% of cervical spine injuries in children. Another study showed that of 42 children with spinal injuries, almost 50% involved the atlas or axis, or both.[12] Fractures of the odontoid process with atlantoaxial dislocations and subluxations, and fractures of the neural arch of the axis are the most common injuries seen in pediatric patients.[13]

Interestingly, there can be an atraumatic atlantoaxial subluxation called Grisel's syndrome, described in 1930 by Grisel.[14] In this syndrome, spontaneous subluxation of the atlas occurs on the axis sec-

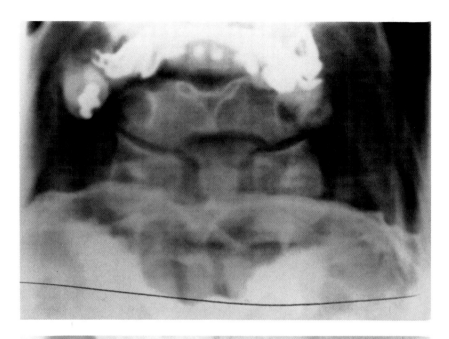

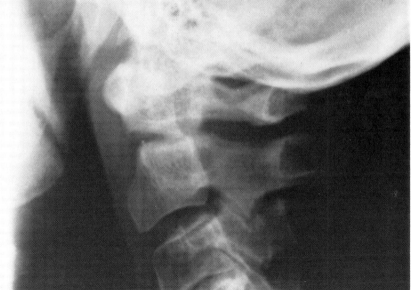

FIG. 7-4. Radiograph of os odontoideum demonstrated in odontoid view.

ondary to an inflammatory response. This usually results from an upper respiratory infection with soft tissue inflammation of the neck and throat causing spontaneous hyperemic subluxation from softening and distension of the ligaments and capsular structures at the atlantoaxial joint. With this, excessive rotation of C_1 on C_2 is allowed with resultant locking of the facets. Other causes have included rheumatoid disease, upper respiratory and throat infections, and tuberculosis.

Children with this syndrome usually have slight to severe neck pain and persistent torticollis. Treatment of the aggravating condition is necessary, as well as reduction of the subluxation. Postreduction use of a soft collar may help alleviate symptoms. In some patients, cervical traction and surgical correction have been indicated.

Radiologic evaluation of this syndrome may be difficult because of the rotary deformity. Radiologic views, therefore, should include a true lateral view of the C_1 to C_2 joint to evaluate the degree of anterior displacement of the atlas on the axis.[15]

Odontoid fractures caused by trauma usually occur at the subdental synchondrosis. Allen and Ferguson,[10] in their review of the literature, found no documentation of apical fractures of the odontoid process. When suspected on x-ray, the odontoid, when fractured, tends to angulate anteriorly with regard to the surrounding structures. Prevertebral swelling may help identify the fracture.

It is important to document this type of fracture for two reasons. First, the fracture usually occurs at the cartilaginous areas and separation of growth centers where growth disturbances can occur. The second is because of Steel's Rule of Thirds,[16] which is that the cervical canal at C_1 is occupied one third by the cord, one third by the odontoid, and one third by free space. Displacement of the odontoid, therefore, may lead to compression of the spinal cord at the level of C_1 to C_2, the cervicomedullary segment.

Atlanto-occiput lesions occur infrequently and are rarely seen because this situation is usually fatal. This injury causes damage to the cervicomedullary spinal cord segment, vertebral and spinal arteries, and usually intracranial injuries. This injury is not seen commonly on x-ray because of spontaneous reduction. The mechanism of injury is probably the result of the large head of the child continuing forward over the craniovertebral junction, with resulting dislocation and subsequent reduction.

Common lesions that occur at C_1 to C_2 or C_2 to C_3 segments are caused by ligamentous disruption or pedicle fractures. Damage to these structures is a result of rotation, flexion, extension, or a combination of any of these mechanisms. Radiographs should be evaluated for subluxation (remembering that a 3- to 4-mm movement of one superior vertebra over inferior vertebra may be normal in a child), prevertebral swelling, and definitive evidence of fracture such as fracture lines or avulsions.

Subluxation and pseudosubluxation may be difficult to differentiate, therefore, certain clues may help. Did the child sustain sufficient trauma for an injury? Are there symptoms despite adequate conservative therapy? Do the films suggest spinal trauma that would be associated with subluxation, such as ossification of the posterior longitudinal ligament or evidence of avulsion fractures of the vertebral body or spinous processes? Does the lower cervical spine gradually develop a compensatory lordosis? Does the subluxation fail to correct with extension?[17]

The soft tissue space in a cooperative child should not be more than 5 mm anterior to C_3.[18] Remember that a screaming, agitated child and expiration may affect the soft tissue space.

Avulsions may not be seen well on x-ray because of the large amount of cartilaginous tissue. If part of the ossified vertebra is also avulsed, this may make it more apparent on x-ray. There should be no open growth plates in the spine after eight years of age,[17] but secondary ossification centers at transverse and spinous processes may persist.

Fractures of the vertebral body occur commonly at C_5 and C_6, with wedge fractures accounting for over 60% and teardrop or burst fractures, 12%.[1] Injuries to the lower cervical spine (C_4 to C_7) are rare. Most commonly, this area of the spine is involved in breech deliveries with the infant's head hyperextended in utero—the "star gazing fetus." Many of these injuries are fatal at birth.

Use of the "posterior cervical line" has been described by Harris and Edeiken-Monroe[19] as a way to differentiate subluxation of C_1 to C_3 from pseudosubluxation. This line helps differentiate whether C_2 displacement is physiologic versus traumatic, on the basis of the posterior laminar line (PLL) of C_2. The posterior cervical line is an imaginary line extending from the PLL of the atlas to the PLL of C_3. In neutral position on a lateral x-ray, the PLL of C_2 lies on or 1 mm anterior or posterior to the PLL. If the axis is intact, the entire unit of C_1 to C_3 moves as a unit; therefore, the unit of C_1 to C_3 forms its own PLL.

With normal flexion, the body of C_2 moves anterior with respect to C_3; therefore, the PLL of C_2 moves 1 to 3 mm anterior to the PLL of the unit. In normal extension, the intact axis will move posteriorly, and its PLL may be 1 to 3 mm posterior to the PLL of the unit.

These observations can also be used for the vertebral bodies of C_2 and C_3 in the neutral, flexed, and extended positions and help show that the anterior and posterior aspect of these vertebrae are intact.

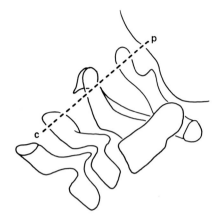

FIG. 7-5. A line drawn from the posterior laminar line (PLL) of C_1 to the PLL of C_3. In a normal condition on a true lateral view C_2 can be 1 mm anterior or posterior of the posterior canal line. This is "pseudosubluxation."

When the above guidelines are met, they help rule out traumatic spondylolisthesis, especially of the axis.[19] Because of the use of the PLL, Harris and Edeiken-Monroe[19] argue against the use of flexion and extension views in cervical spine fractures in children (Fig. 7-5).

Congenital lesions must also be considered. Patients with Down's syndrome have an increased atlanto-dental interval secondary to laxity of the transverse atlanto-ligament.[13]

Klippel-Feil syndrome includes patients with congenital fusion of two or more cervical vertebrae. These patients frequently have genitourinary, neurologic, cardiopulmonary, and auditory involvement. Often, there is a triad that consists of low posterior hairline, short neck, and limitation of motion of the head and neck, usually in the lateral direction. These patients may also have facial asymmetry, torticollis, and webbing of the neck.[20]

The syndrome is important because a child or adolescent may arrive at the ED after a minor traumatic event with signs and symptoms of neurologic injury that may be complications of this syndrome. Hypermobility of the vertebrae caused by ligamentous and capsular stretching, arthritic changes with disc space and spinal canal narrowing, and fusion of the vertebral bodies can contribute to spinal column and spinal cord damage.

Recognition of spinal column fractures in children is important not only neurologically, but also because of their effect on the spinal column itself. Injury to the spinal column may lead to unstable malalignment of the spine with disruption of the ligaments and subsequent deformity, which usually results in scoliosis or kyphosis of the involved area. This is especially true in the thoracic and cervicothoracic spine. These deformities can be treated with braces or surgery involving fusion techniques.

In addition to the obvious paraplegia or tetraplegia, other multisystem problems can occur from cervical spine injury. Some intrathoracic problems that can occur include flail chest, pulmonary and/or cardiac contusion, and tension pneumothorax; abdominal problems include fractures of the spleen and liver, pelvic fractures with retroperitoneal hematoma, injuries to the pancreas and duodenum, and so forth. The ED physician must be aware of these potential problems because they may be present when the patient arrives. Some of the complications may occur later in the rehabilitation period, but early preventative measures can help decrease the incidence of their appearance in these patients.

The respiratory system may suffer early from respiratory insufficiency in the case of a high cord lesion, which can be managed with early airway management. Later, atelectasis and pneumonia may occur.

The gastrointestinal system will suffer paralytic ileus and gastric dilatation that can be controlled with early nasogastric tube placement. Gastrointestinal bleeding and ulcerations may develop later.

Initially, there will be urinary retention, which can be minimized with bladder catheterization to prevent overdistension. An intermittent catheterization program, as soon as possible, will help restore bladder tone and decrease the incidence of urinary infection. Chronically, calcium urolithiasis with hydronephrosis may develop.

Hypercalcemia and osteoporosis can occur because of resorption from bone. This hypercalcemia is a precipitating factor in the development of urolithiasis. Decubitus ulcers may appear during convalescence. Deep vein thrombosis may form in paralyzed lower extremities and lead to pulmonary embolization.

Septicemia is a disastrous, long-term consequence as a complication of bacterial colonization and infection of the lungs, bladder, and decubitus. Prevention of these problems, therefore, may be augmented by early intervention in the spinal cord-injured patient in the ED.[21,22]

REFERENCES

1. Kewalramani LS: Spinal cord injury in children, in Calenoff L (ed): *Radiology of Spinal Cord Injury.* St. Louis, CV Mosby Co., 1981, pp 503–540.
2. Caffey J: The whiplash-shaken infant syndrome. *Pediatrics* 1974;54(4):734.
3. Swischuck LE: Spine and spinal cord trauma in the battered child syndrome. *Radiology* 1969;92:733.

4. Ahmann PA, Smith SA, Schwartz JF, et al: Spinal cord infarction due to minor trauma in children. *Neurology* 1975;25:301–307.

5. Burke DC: Traumatic spinal paralysis in children. *Paraplegia* 1974;11:268–276.

6. Vigoroux RP, Baurance C, Choux M, et al: Injuries of the cervical spine in children. *Neurochirurgia* 1968;14:689–702.

7. Cattell HS, Filtzer DL: Pseudosubluxation and other normal variations in the cervical spine of children. *J Bone Joint Surg* 1965;47A:1295–1309.

8. Sullivan CR, Bruwer AJ, Harris LE: Hypermobility of the cervical spine in children: A pitfall in the diagnosis of cervical dislocations. *Am J Surg* 1958;95:636–640.

9. Yashon D. *Spinal Injury,* New York, Appleton-Century-Crofts, 1978.

10. Allen BL, Ferguson RL: Cervical spine trauma in children, in Bradford DS, Hensinger RM (eds): *The Pediatric Spine,* New York, Thieme, Inc., 1985, pp 89–104.

11. Hause M, Hoshino R, Omata S, et al: Cervical spine injuries in children. *Fukushima J Med Sci* 1974;20:114.

12. Hubbard DD: Injuries of the spine in children and adolescents. *Clin Orthop* 1974;100:56–65.

13. Sherk HH, Schut L, Lane JM: Fractures and dislocations of the cervical spine in children. *Orthop Clin North Am* 1976;7(3):593–604.

14. Grisel P: Enucleation de l'atlas et torticollis nasopharyngien. *Presse Med* 1930;38:50.

15. Lippman RK: Arthropathy due to adjacent inflammation. *J Bone Joint Surg* 1953;35A(4).

16. Steel HH: Anatomical and mechanical consideration of the atlantoaxial articulation: Proceedings of the American Orthopedic Association. *J Bone Joint Surg* 1968;50A:1481.

17. Fielding JW: Cervical spine injuries in children, in The Cervical Research Society (eds): *The Cervical Spine.* Philadelphia, JB Lippincott Co, 1983, pp 268–281.

18. Denton JR: Trauma and the adolescent spine, in Keim HS (ed): *The Adolescent Spine.* New York, Springer-Verlag, 1976, pp 63–95.

19. Harris JH, Edeiken-Monroe B: *The Radiology of Acute Cervical Trauma,* ed. 2, Baltimore, Williams and Wilkins, 1987.

20. Hensinger RN: Orthopedic problems of the shoulder and neck. *Pediatr Clin North Am* 1977;24(4):889–902.

21. Babcock JL: Spinal injuries in children. *Pediatr Clin North Am* 1975;22(2):487–500.

22. Hoffman HJ, Hendrick EB, Humphreys RP: Spinal cord injuries, in Surgical Staff of the Hospital for Sick Children (eds): *Care for the Injured Child.* Toronto, Williams and Wilkins Co, 1975, pp 78–87.

8

NORMAN E. MCSWAIN, JR.

Acute Management

PRINCIPLES

In the management of every medical problem, major *principles* must be addressed, but people *prefer* to accomplish these principles in multiple ways. So it is with the management of possible cervical spine injuries within the prehospital area and in the Emergency Department (ED). To stabilize any fracture properly, the joint above and below the fracture must be immobilized. The joint above a cervical spine fracture is between C_1 and the skull, and the joint below the cervical spine fracture is between C_7 and T_1. Proper immobilization of the entire spine requires immobilization of the last joint of the spine, including the lumbosacral joint. To stabilize this joint, the pelvis must be fixed. Correct management of a spinal fracture, therefore, is to place the patient on a backboard with the pelvis, chest or abdomen, and head immobilized (Fig. 8-1). It is incorrect management to immobilize the head alone and have the patient simply lie on the backboard. If the patient becomes unruly, disoriented, or for any other reason rolls to the side, with the head restrained, movement of the rest of the spine will put major stress and strain on the cervical spine. This can produce severe damage to the cord when an unstable fracture is present.

Helmet Removal

Although many states have no mandatory helmet laws, others do. In those states that do not have mandatory helmet laws, some riders

105

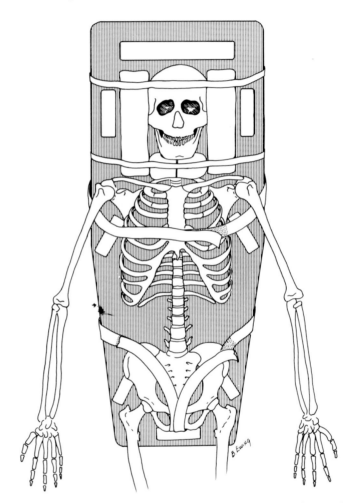

FIG. 8-1.   Immobilization of the "joint above and the joint below." The possible fractures require that the entire spine be immobilized, which requires immobilization of the skull, thorax, and pelvis. Immobilization lacking the above will allow some portion of the spine to have free movement.

wish to protect themselves from head injury by wearing one. Most helmets that are effective fit fairly tight to the head (including football helmets). It is important that the cervical spine is maintained in a neutral position when these helmets are removed from patients. This can be accomplished easily if certain basic principles are remembered.

1. Immobilization of the cervical spine is maintained by immobilization of the head.

2. The helmet must be expanded laterally to clear the ears.
3. Anterior rotation of the helmet is required to clear the occiput.
4. A full facial coverage helmet cannot be removed without first removing glasses (if worn).
5. It is not necessary to cut or saw the helmet, simply remove it. The basic steps are:
    A. Immobilization is established by placing one hand in front of the neck with pressure on each mandibular angulus through the thumb and index finger. The second hand is placed behind the neck on the occiput (Fig. 8-2).
    B. The helmet is expanded laterally to clear the ears (Fig. 8-3), and rotated forward to clear the occiput (Fig. 8-4).
    C. After removal, in-line immobilization is reestablished from above (Figs. 8-4 and 8-5).

Proper immobilization of the head also requires placing the neck within 11° of its normal neutral position. The scapula, posterior muscles of the thorax, and kyphosis of the thoracic spine produce a more anterior position of the head, directly in line with the posterior aspect portion of the torso as a person ages. A child has a flat posterior thoracic

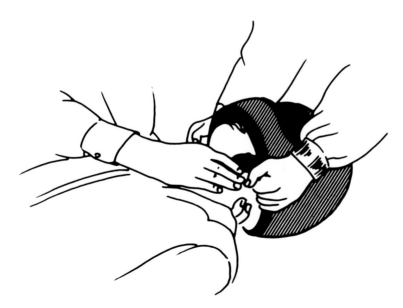

FIG. 8-2. Removal of a helmet (motorcycle, football, or other) is achieved by placing in-line immobilization from below. One hand in front of the neck on the angulus of the mandible and the other on the posterior skull. (Reprinted with permission of the American College of Surgeons/Committee on Trauma.)

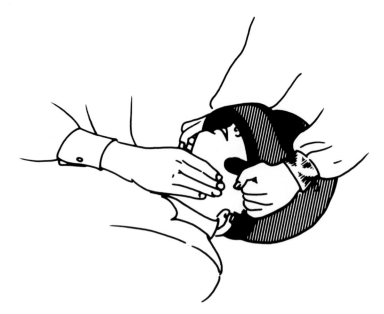

FIG. 8-3. The helmet is expended laterally to clear the ears. (Reprinted with permission of the American College of Surgeons/Committee on Trauma.)

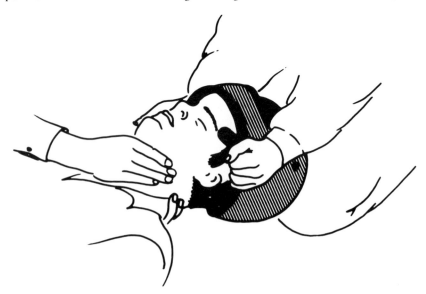

FIG. 8-4. The helmet is rotated anteriorly to clear the occiput. Some slight anterior movement of the neck may be necessary to get the helmet completely clear of the occiput. This movement should be as minimal as possible and should be done gently and slowly. (Reprinted with permission of the American College of Surgeons/Committee on Trauma.)

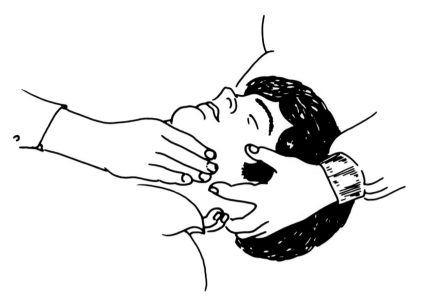

FIG. 8-5. After the helmet is removed, the hands should be replaced from above so that adequate immobilization to a backboard can then be completed. (Reprinted with permission of the American College of Surgeons/Committee on Trauma.)

wall and a mobile thoracic spine. If placed directly on a spine board, the child's head is in severe hyperflexion, which not only places the cervical spine in a precarious position, but may also compromise the airway (Fig. 8-6). As the aging process continues, the C_7-T_1 junction becomes more anterior. The child will require padding beneath the scapulae (Fig. 8-7), the young adult no padding, and the elderly person padding beneath the occiput, to maintain the correct neutral position (Fig. 8-8).

Usually, three pieces of equipment are used for spine immobilization. The long backboard is used both as immobilization and a movement device (Fig. 8-9). The short backboard is used as an immobilization device and an extrication device (Fig. 8-10). Frequently, the patient arrives at the hospital on both the short backboard used to provide immobilization during the extrication process, and a long backboard used for movement of the patient. It is acceptable to leave both devices in place while the lateral cervical spine and other appropriate x-rays are obtained.

The cervical collar is a device used to provide assistance in stabilizing the patient to the backboard. The straps to immobilize the head are frequently brought across the cervical collar to provide lateral sta-

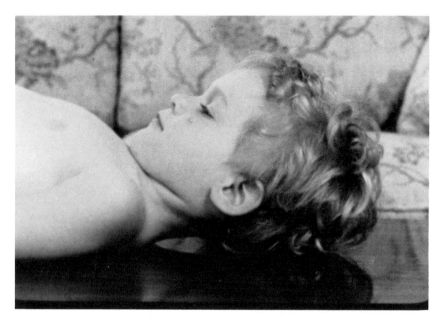

FIG. 8-6. The very posterior location of C_7-T_2 in a child produces hyperflexion when placed supine on a backboard.

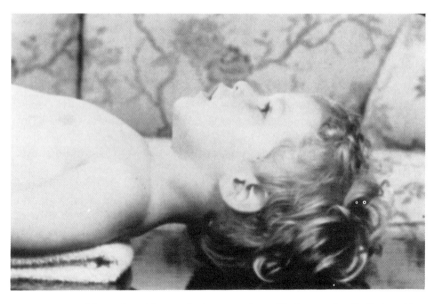

FIG. 8-7. Padding placed beneath the scapulae will elevate the C_7-T_1 junction to allow immobilization of the spine in the neutral position in the child.

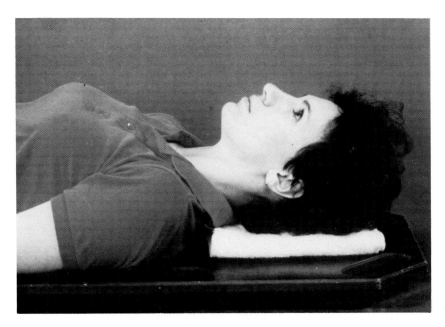

FIG. 8-8. As age progresses, the C_7-T_1 junction is located more anteriorly. Neutral position in the adult requires varying amounts of padding beneath the skull to maintain the neutral position of the cervical spine.

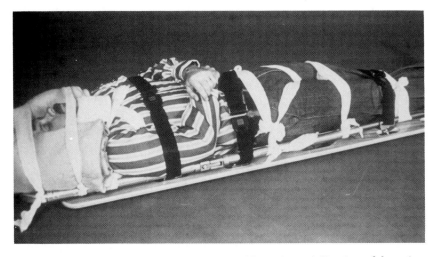

FIG. 8-9. The long backboard provides total bony immobilization of the spine, as well as the long bones. It is also an excellent device for moving the patient both on and off of stretchers, x-ray tables, etc.

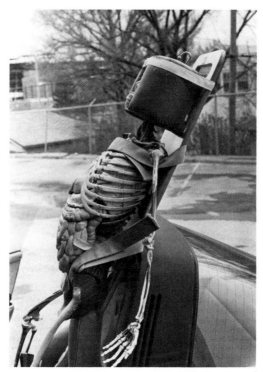

FIG. 8-10. The short backboard, which fits behind the patient, provides a means for removal from the vehicle while maintaining immobilization of the entire spine.

bilization, however, the cervical collar should not be used alone as an immobilization device. The soft cervical collar provides almost no immobilization, whereas hard collars, such as the "Stiff Neck®" and "Philadelphia Collar®," provide approximately 50% immobilization in the three critical movements of anterior-posterior, lateral, and rotation. Used in combination with the backboard, the cervical collar is a helpful device and is useful for cervical spines.

Immobilization of the pelvis is straightforward and is done with the long backboard by straps across the pelvis and thighs. Immobilization of the chest and abdomen is also a simple technique because a strap secured directly across the chest or abdomen can provide such immobilization (Fig. 8-11).

The head, however, is much more complicated. It would be simple enough if a strap was placed around the chin and head (Fig. 8-12). Such a technique, however, is extremely dangerous because the force to prevent head movement is provided at the mandible to the skull via

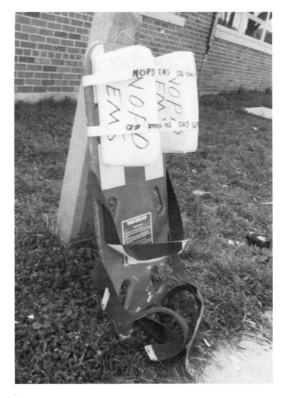

FIG. 8-11. Strapping to immobilize the pelvis consists of a strap around each leg across the wing of the ilium and through the crotch. The chest strap crosses below the arms and above the epigastrium.

tight approximation of the molars. Such approximation prevents opening of the mouth. If the patient vomits, which is common in trauma situations, aspiration is almost guaranteed. Aspiration of gastric contents increases the mortality rate to 80%. This, added to complications of trauma, severely compromises an already precarious situation.

Airway Management

Management of the airway in a patient with a possible cervical spine fracture requires that the cervical spine not be moved during these maneuvers. Although this seems complicated, it simply requires two people to establish the airway rather than one, and that the tongue is the most common source of airway obstruction. The tongue is attached to the mandible. Movement of the mandible forward will also bring

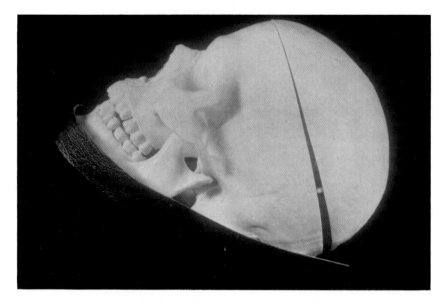

FIG. 8-12. A chin strap placed across the chin to immobilize the head requires pressure directed from the mandible through the lower molars to the upper molars to hold the skull against the backboard. The jaw is thus held closed. If the patient vomits, vomitus into the closed mouth can be aspirated into the lungs.

the tongue forward. The jaw lift, jaw thrust, and chin lift maneuvers are simple means of opening the airway without compromise of the cervical spine position.

More advanced airway maneuvers, such as insertion of the endotracheal tube, require one person to immobilize the head and one to insert the tube. This is best done from below by reaching across the chest with one hand and placing the palms of the hands over either ear. Medial pressure immobilizes the head and cervical spine (the arm reaching across the chest provides immobilization of the joint below the fracture).

Placing the head in the sniffing position hyperextends the cervical spine at C_2-C_3 and hyperflexes it at C_5-C_6 (Fig. 8-13). To avoid these, the head is maintained in the neutral position. Visualization of the trachea and larynx is accomplished by anterior and candid movement of the mandible. Although this can be done with either type of laryngoscope blade, I prefer the straight blade.

Pads are placed on either side of the patient's head and strapped

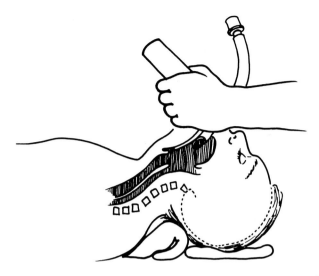

FIG. 8-13. The sniffing position hyperextends the neck at C_2-C_3 and hyperflexes it at C_5-C_6. It should not be used for endotracheal tube placement in the trauma patient. For insertion of the tube in a patient with a possible cervical spine fracture, the neck should be held in the neutral position while the mandible is moved forward to visualize the larynx. (Reprinted from the Prehospital Trauma Life Support Course by permission of Emergency Training® 1988.)

tightly to the backboard to prevent head motion (Fig. 8-14). Several commercially available backboards reduce neck motion to a minimum. When using the long backboards without such immobilization pads, other steps must be taken. A rolled blanket placed in a horseshoe-shape over the patient's head not only provides lateral stability, but also can be folded and slid behind the head to provide padding for the neutral position (Fig. 8-15). Lateral padding can be provided using intravenous bags or sand bags. In general, sand bags should not be used in ambulance transportation because of the extra weight and lateral stress that can be placed on the head if the strapping is loosened.

When moving a patient before the backboard has been applied, or when necessary to move the patient without the backboard, the spine should be moved in one unit and not be allowed to turn or angulate. Several methods can be used to accomplish such a maneuver, but all require the coordinated effort of at least four people. The team leader places his hands over the ears of the patient so that direct, positive control of the head and cervical spine is obtained and maintained.

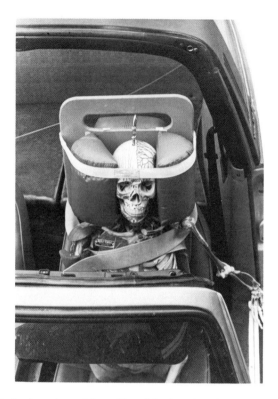

FIG. 8-14. Pads placed on either side of the head and strapped tightly against the skull prevent rotation, flexion, extension, and lateral flexion and allow access to the airway. (Reprinted from the Prehospital Trauma Life Support Course by permission of Emergency Training® 1988).

The second mover (or two movers if available) is responsible for the thoracic spine. Placement of the support is beneath the shoulders and lower thoracic vertebrae. The next person (or two people if available) is responsible for lifting the hips and maintaining the in-line stability of the lumbar spine. The last mover assumes the responsibility of the legs to assure the pelvis does not tilt upward or downward and produce angulation of the lumbar spine.

On occasion, a patient will arrive at the ED whose history of trauma or presenting signs (blunt injury above the clavicle, head at a peculiar angle, supporting head with hand) indicates the possibility of a cervical fracture. Appropriate precautions must be taken to prevent neurologic complications of this injury.

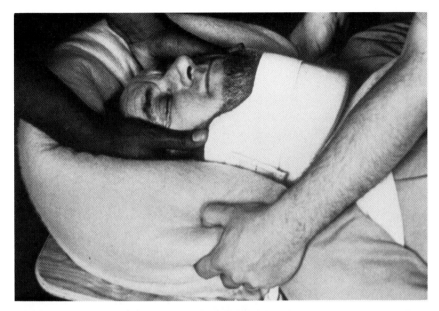

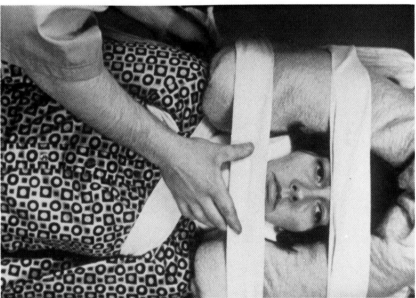

FIG. 8-15. When other means of cervical padding are not available or are unsatisfactory, a "horse collar" (a) made of a rolled blanket provides excellent immobilization. It is strapped against the head with strong 2" or 3" tape (b). (Reprinted from the Prehospital Trauma Life Support Course by permission of Emergency Training® 1988.)

Traction, in general, is not used for management of cervical spine injuries in the initial phase of evaluation because it tends to distract unstable segments. Application of cervical tongs for the definitive treatment of cervical injuries is appropriate. The exact positioning to ensure proper angle of pull and the correct amount of weight necessary to accomplish unlocking of facets or other cervical problems, however, is beyond the scope of this text.

JORGE A. MARTINEZ

Self-Evaluation

This chapter consists of five case presentations and questions regarding evaluation of the cervical spine. They have been included as an informal type of self-evaluation in the approach to injuries of the cervical spine. These cases will allow the reader to use some of the information in the previous chapters when answering the questions. They are, however, in no way meant to be inclusive of all the material in the book—this would necessitate a separate book in itself.

CASE 1

A 36-year-old male was brought into the Emergency Department (ED) after being hit by a train. The patient was found in a ditch next to the train tracks by the Emergency Medical Technicians. The patient was lying in a puddle of water with an obvious fracture of the right forearm and left lower leg. There was a large abrasion to the forehead. The patient was responsive to vocal and painful stimuli and smelled of alcohol. He was transported on a long spine board with immobilization of his neck. An intravenous (IV) line of lactated Ringer's and oxygen (3 L/min) nasal cannula were also started.

Upon arrival in the ED, the Advanced Trauma Life Support protocol recommended by the American College of Surgeons was initiated: 1) primary survey—including airway, breathing, circulation as-

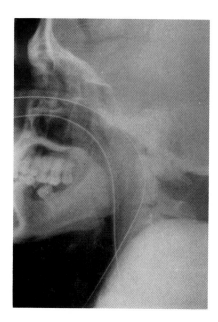 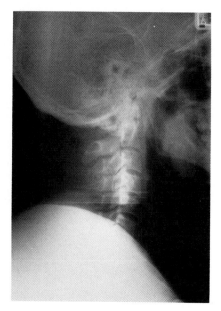

sessment, disability (physical and neurologic), and expose (undress); 2) resuscitation—including IV fluids, oxygen, cardiac monitor, direct pressure to bleeding sites, and nasogastric tube and Foley catheters if not contraindicated; 3) secondary survey—including a head-to-toe physical examination and neurologic evaluation; and 4) definitive treatment.

Examination of the patient showed open fractures of the right forearm and left lower leg. The head, chest, abdomen, and pelvis were normal except for abrasions to the forehead. Examination of the neck disclosed diffuse tenderness posteriorly along its entire length. No open lesions, bony step-offs, or deformities were found. The neurologic examination was normal.

Questions:

a. What do the cervical spine films show?
b. What other diagnostic study could have been done to confirm the diagnosis?

Answers:

a. The cross-table lateral view shows a nonunion of the dorsal arch of the first cervical vertebra. The unjoined ends are smooth and rounded, whereas fractured ends would be sharp and jagged. Additionally, no free bits of bone are located between the open ends. A diagnosis of congenital nonunion of the dorsal arch of C_1 was made.

b. A computed tomography (CT) scan of the cervical spine is a rapid and specific method that can be used to evaluate the cervical spine. This procedure confirmed the diagnosis and ruled out any other cervical spine injuries.

CASE 2

A 27-year-old female was brought to the ED after being involved in an automobile accident. At the scene the patient was unconscious, and it was noted that her head had hit the windshield causing a "bullseye" effect. She had a laceration to the forehead, but no other obvious injuries were noted. The patient was extricated by Emergency Medical Technicians and transferred to the hospital on a long spine board, with cervical spine immobilization and an IV of lactated Ringer's.

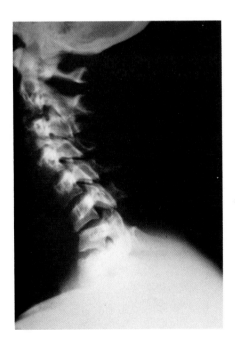

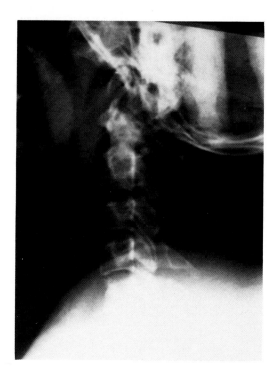

Upon arrival in the ED, the patient remained unconscious. Her vital signs were stable. Trauma evaluation, as recommended by the American College of Surgeons Advanced Trauma Life Support, only disclosed the laceration of the scalp. Neurologic examination was unable to be performed thoroughly because of the patient's level of consciousness. She did, however, wince with painful stimuli. No spontaneous movements or withdrawal from pain were found. The anal sphincter tone was intact.

X-rays of the skull, cervical spine, and chest were taken. The x-rays of the skull and chest were normal. The films of the cervical spine were repeated.

Questions:

a. Why were the cervical spine films repeated?
b. What was the problem found on the subsequent films?

Answers:

a. The cervical spine films had to be repeated because all seven cervical vertebrae were not seen in the originals. All seven cervical vertebrae must be seen before the film can be considered adequate. If the lateral film cannot visualize all seven vertebrae, the "swimmer's" view should be used.

b. The repeat cervical spine films indicate a C_6 on C_7 subluxation. This was found only after a complete cervical spine film was obtained. If this had been missed, the patient could have suffered irreparable damage from spinal cord injury secondary to the unstable cervical spine segments.

CASE 3

A 19-year-old male was involved in a motorcycle accident, causing him to be thrown from his motorcycle and land on his side. He denied any loss of consciousness but complained of severe pain in the upper neck posteriorly. He denied any numbness or tingling of the extremities and had no problems with motion or sensation. He was wearing a helmet while riding the motorcycle.

The patient was transported to the ED on a long spine board. The cervical collar had been applied simultaneously with proper removal of the helmet. An IV of lactated Ringer's was started. The patient remained alert and conscious during the transfer.

Evaluation in the ED followed the American College of Surgeons Advanced Trauma Life Support protocol. The physical examination disclosed multiple abrasions to the extremities and chest. Severe tenderness was noted upon palpation of the upper neck posteriorly, but no open lesions, bony step-offs, or deformities. Examination of the head, face, chest, abdomen, pelvis, and extremities, other than the noted abrasions, was normal. The neurologic examination was normal.

X-rays of the chest and cervical spine were performed. The chest films were normal.

Questions:

a. What is the condition in the lateral cervical spine view?

b. What other diagnostic studies could be done to confirm the diagnosis?

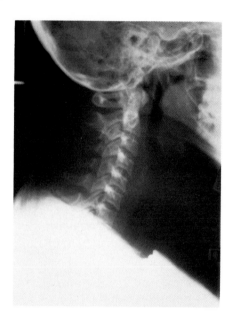

Answers:

a. The lateral cervical spine view indicates a linear fracture through the lateral aspect of the dorsal arch of C_1. It is nondisplaced. No odontoid deviation or prevertebral swelling is noted.

b. Other studies that could be used to confirm the diagnosis are: 1) an open-mouth odontoid view, which may show the fracture line through the atlas; 2) tomograms of the suspicious area of C_1; and 3) CT scan for planar views of the first cervical vertebra.

CASE 4

A 34-year-old male was involved in an altercation. During the incident he was kicked in the back of the head while lying on the floor. He claimed that he immediately felt weak and dizzy and developed numbness and tingling in both of his arms and legs. He denied any loss of consciousness or previous episodes of numbness or tingling.

He was transported to the ED on a long spine board with cervical immobilization. A complete history and physical examination

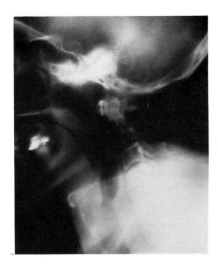
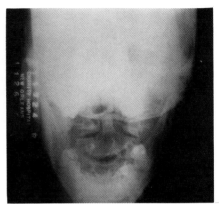

were done as recommended by the American College of Surgeons Advanced Trauma Life Support protocol. Positive findings indicated a large hematoma to the posterior scalp and multiple bruises and abrasions to the face, neck, extremities, chest, and abdomen. Examination of the neck was negative for deformities or bony step-offs. Diffuse tenderness and bruising of the neck were noted. The neurologic examination disclosed decreased strength of the upper and lower extremities with normal sensation, but persistent numbness and tingling. Anal sphincter tone was intact. Vital signs were stable. Appropriate x-rays were taken, with only the cervical spine films demonstrating pathologic findings.

Questions:

a. What pathologic findings did the cervical spine films show?
b. What is the classification of this type of fracture?

Answers:

a. The cervical spine film indicates an odontoid fracture, Type III. The open-mouth odontoid view is best for demonstrating the odontoid fracture. Most odontoid fractures can also be seen on the lateral cervical spine views.
b. Three types of odontoid fractures have been described. Type I is an avulsion fracture of the tip of the odontoid. It is a rare type of fracture that is relatively stable. Type II odontoid fractures are

limited to the odontoid process and usually involve its inferior aspect. These types of fractures are unstable and have the potential to cause spinal cord injury. Type III odontoid fractures are fractures of the superior aspect of the body of the axis. It, therefore, involves the entire odontoid process and the part of the axis that attaches to the odontoid process. This fracture is also unstable and can cause damage of the spinal cord. Both Types II and III fractures can be caused by hyperextension or hyperflexion. They are also usually associated with prevertebral swelling, and because they are unstable, can cause mild to severe spinal cord injuries.[1]

CASE 5

A three-year-old male child was brought to the ED after having fallen out of his bunkbed, approximately 4 feet. The mother stated that the child landed on his back when he fell. The child was found to be unresponsive to vocal or painful stimuli, with a distended abdomen and shallow, rapid respirations. He was immediately "log rolled" onto a long spine board and the cervical spine immobilized. An airway was established, while protecting the cervical spine, using high-flow oxygen. Two peripheral IVs of lactated Ringer's were also begun.

A complete physical examination was begun using the American College of Surgeons Advanced Trauma Life Support protocol. It disclosed a large hematoma to the posterior aspect of the scalp and distended abdomen with minimal bowel sounds and guarding. Neurologically, the child remained quiet and unresponsive to vocal stimuli, but did respond to painful stimuli with grimacing and whimpering. Pupillary reactions were normal, as was anal sphincter tone. Deep tendon reflexes were decreased diffusely. The vital signs were tachycardia with hypotension, which responded to boluses of IV fluids. A diagnosis of acute abdomen was made and immediate abdominal exploration was planned. A lateral cervical spine film was done to evaluate the cervical spine for injury.

Questions:

a. What is the diagnosis based on the cervical spine films?
b. What considerations need to be undertaken when reviewing the cervical spine films of children under eight years old?

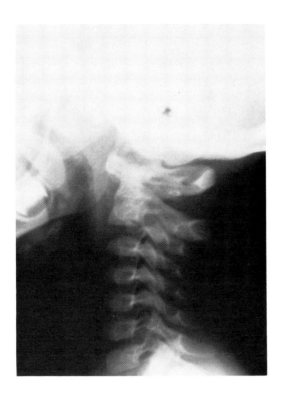

Answers:

a. The film shows "pseudosubluxation" or physiologic subluxation of the cervical spine. This phenomenon occurs most commonly at the C_2 to C_3 junction. Pseudosubluxation can be differentiated from true subluxation by using the C_1 to C_2 to C_3 posterior line. It is done by drawing a line from the cortex of the posterior arch of C_1 to the cortex of the posterior arch of the third cervical vertebra. The anatomic relationship is normal between C_1 to C_3 if this line passes through or just behind the anterior cortex of the posterior arch of C_2, or if it touches or is within 1 mm of the cortex of C_2.[2]

b. A child's cervical spine varies from that of an adult in several ways. First, because of the laxity of the transverse atlantal ligament, there can be a greater motion between the axis and the atlas; therefore, the interval between the atlas and odontoid process can be from 3 to 5 mm. This interval is 3 mm or less in adults. Second, the ligamentous laxity of the atlas and axis, and incomplete ossification of the distal aspect of the odontoid, allow as much as two thirds of the atlas to appear above the tip of the odontoid process when seen in the lateral projection. Third, the laxity of the ligaments and shallowness of the interfacetal joints at C_2 to C_3 and C_3 to C_4 allow the physiologic subluxation, which can be identified in lateral cervical films. Fourth, because of the maleability of the prevertebral soft tissues, a "pseudomass" can be seen on lateral projections, which is a result of physiologic prevertebral soft tissue expansion that occurs commonly with expiration. This can be differentiated from true prevertebral swelling by taking the cervical spine film with the neck slightly hyperextended and during inspiration. Pathologic prevertebral swelling, such as that caused by an expanding hematoma or retropharyngeal abscess will not disappear with inspiration.[3]

REFERENCES

1. Harris JH, Edeiken-Monroe B (eds): Injuries of diverse or poorly understood mechanisms. *The Radiology of Acute Cervical Spine Trauma,* ed. 2. Baltimore, Williams and Wilkins, 1987, pp 220–279.
2. Frame SB, Hendrickson MF: Problem: Pediatric cervical spine injuries. *Emerg Med* 1987;November, pp 47–51.
3. Harris JH: Radiographic evaluation of spinal trauma. *Orthop Clin North Am* 1986;17(1):75–86.

INDEX